ONCE AND FOR ALL

BIG GOD † BIG FREE ®

ONCE AND FOR ALL

A Faith–Based, Biblically Principled Approach to Eradicating Addictions

Michelle Behrenwald

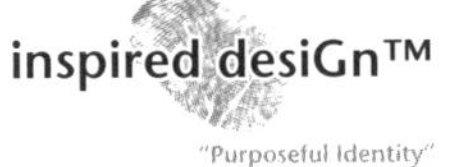

Scripture version permissions:

Most frequently used version: NIV

Other versions used: AMPLIFIED, KJV, MESSAGE, NKJV, NLT

ACKNOWLEDGEMENTS

Kudos and the applause of heaven to the "Living Witnesses"—proof of God's Truth—that Jesus Paid the Price for our Salvation, Freedom, Healing and Restoration and that God is a Big God. Your testimonials are inspiring examples and your words of encouragement will make a difference! Journey on in Freedom—your crown awaits (James 1:12).

Special Appreciation, Gratitude and Thanksgiving to:

- ☐ My Father and Mother, Larry and Kay Behrenwald and my dear friends Pastor Alex and Laura Chavez for the mega amounts of guidance, support and coaching. You loved me, encouraged me, stepped out with me as I began working with the Lord in His Freedom ministry and trained me spiritually in God's Truth—Thank You!

- ☐ My brother, Jim Behrenwald, who taught me to do what I love, to keep going no matter what anyone says and no matter the odds or the cost.

- ☐ Valerie Sall for the wonderful root illustrations, spiritual encouragement and friendship along the way.

- ☐ Trish Konieczny, my editor, for her invaluable professional assistance and support. She ensured excellence in this piece of work.

Most importantly, thank you to the Lord God Almighty, my Heavenly Father (Papa), for giving us this way to live full and free lives here on earth as it is in heaven. Thank you Jesus Christ — you paid the price and praise you Holy Spirit for you confirm the truth with your presence and power. God is a triune God, to Him be the Glory and Honor. Today, I experience great joy in being His child and being part of His ministry to others.

Big God†Big Free!®

CONTENTS

BIG GOD†BIG FREE®

INTRODUCTION

If we consider the unblushing promises of reward and the staggering nature of the rewards promised in the Gospels, it would seem that our Lord finds our desires not too strong, but too weak. We are half-hearted creatures, fooling about with drink and sex and ambition when infinite joy is offered us, like an ignorant child who wants to go on making mud pies in a slum because he cannot imagine what is meant by the offer of a holiday at the sea. We are far too easily pleased.

C. S. Lewis

The goal of this book is to provide readers with the truth—the kind of truth that will set them free, as Jesus Christ promised: "And you shall know the truth, and the truth shall make you free" (John 8:32, NKJV). An addiction of any type is a form of bondage. It controls you and limits you. Picture a dog on a chain. He is outside, so he is somewhat free. However, he is not completely free—he can only go as far as the chain will allow. He can get a running start, but then bam, he is on the ground, stopped by the chain. Addictions are like the chain on the dog. They work the same way, hindering us and preventing us from living the full and abundant life God designed for us. They kill, steal and destroy us and those around us.

The truth, though, is that there is a way out. You can obtain freedom today! The foundation for getting free lies in God's Truth and a faith-based approach. The key is to apply biblically based principles related to eradicating addictions and restoring your heart. This eradication and restoration is based on the life work of Jesus Christ as Lord and Savior and the confirming power of the Holy Spirit. It is His work, not mine. Jesus Christ paid the all-sufficient price on the cross for you—**Once and For All.** Jesus Christ came to rescue, to heal, to restore and to set the captives free. Bondage is the opposite of freedom. God wants you free, **completely free**, as Jesus was completely free. He can take care of any problem, hang-up or habit you have. He said in John 6:63 that the words He spoke—they are spirit and they are life.

THIS BOOK'S BASIS: GOD'S TRUTH WILL SET YOU FREE

This book will allow the readers to increase their understanding and knowledge of the truth, increase their faith, and release the Holy Spirit's power and anointing to eradicate and replace addictions in their life with the love of God. It is different from other worldly methods or processes available today due to the following reasons:

- ☐ It is based on Jesus Christ and the work of the Holy Spirit (it is God-made, not man-made)
- ☐ It eradicates the addiction versus medicating it
- ☐ It deals with the heart/spiritual issues behind the addiction and replaces them with God's love and promises
- ☐ It provides biblically based truths for maintaining freedom versus coping with the problem
- ☐ It is simple and clear
- ☐ There is no condemnation for the addict—just restoration. Jesus never condemns. He came to heal, deliver and restore!
- ☐ It assists the readers up and out of bondage—into their God-given calling and purpose

☐ It emphasizes that today is freedom day—not tomorrow, next week or next year—today!

☐ Big God means Big Free!

I know for a fact that God's word is truth and it works. Personally, I have been set free through it. I also teach a "Free Indeed" series based on these biblical principles, and I have seen them in action. As we minister to individuals with different addictions, the Holy Spirit confirms these truths that set people free. I have seen them applied not only to all kinds of addictions including, smoking, pornography, eating disorders, gambling, anger, fear, drug use, anxiety disorders, and a host of other issues. Whatever has you bound is coming off in Jesus' name!

I want to be clear that this book's intent is not to downplay or disregard other methods or plans that help individuals with addictions. Rather it is to provide a faith-based, biblically principled approach to addiction eradication, replacement and heart restoration. Any method that helps an individual overcome their addiction without countering God's Truth should be viewed in a positive light. I consider all individuals free moral agents, the way God designed us, and I would not want life any other way. I believe that if you freely choose to walk through this process, God will honor and bless your efforts—so read on and get free!

THIS BOOK'S PURPOSE: HELPING YOU GET FREE!

The purpose of this guide is simple—Jesus paid the price for our freedom, so let's get free! Several sections of foundational freedom principles and truths are included; perhaps you already know these in part or in full. They are provided to build and refresh your faith. The goal is to come up and out of that which entangles you and into your God given calling and destiny. This is not Michelle's plan; this is God's plan as He gave it to us in His Word. I am merely one of the megaphones He has chosen to use. He wants you free, and He is a 100 percent kind of God who never changes and never fails.

Please enjoy your reading, and remember, God never condemns you. Rather, He convicts you and desires that you to take His path, a better way to complete freedom today. God loves you. I smoked for over 20 years, and I tried many times to quit but could never sustain it. I never tried it with the truth and power of God, though. His way is different. It gets to the root of the problem. Until the root is removed and replaced, it will only drive you to stay addicted to whatever has you bound or even cause you to find a new addiction to something else. It will never allow you to be satisfied and fulfilled. The good news is that God always provides a way: "God is faithful . . . when you are tempted, He will also provide a way out so that you can stand" (1 Corinthians 10:13, NIV). And what God does, He does forever! I am living proof.

INVITATION AND OPENING PRAYER

I would like to open your reading with the following prayer (please pray this out loud):

> *Heavenly Father, in the name of Jesus, we welcome You to this place and into our lives. Holy Spirit, we ask that You prepare and open our hearts to receive the powerful and living Word of the Lord. Remove any thinking that isn't in agreement with God's ways and open our spiritual eyes and ears to hear and receive. We welcome You to heal, restore and deliver us; to touch our hearts, our minds, our emotions and our bodies today, in the name of Jesus. We thank You, Lord Jesus, for Your death and resurrection. It is Your blood that cleanses us from our unrighteousness and restores us. We speak to fear, anxiety and any enemy forces and render you useless in the name of Jesus. Father, release Your Holy Spirit of Life, Love, Liberty and Adoption to flow freely in our lives from this day forward. Lord, touch each person with Your presence, in the name of Jesus Christ, Amen.*

HOW TO USE THIS BOOK AND ITS COMPANION TOOL KIT

Using this book as a guide, you will gain insight into God's plan for your life. His plan is for you to experience freedom, healing, restoration and fullness of life. When that happens to you, it doesn't mean hard times will no longer come, but it means that you will go through them differently. They will not have the same effect on you that they once did.

Let the information presented in this book help you on your way to eradicating your addictions and experiencing the healing restoration of your heart. Each chapter contains various items that I hope you will find useful. The chapters begin with stories of individuals who have overcome their addictions. While your freedom process won't be exactly like anyone else's, I hope their testimonials will encourage you. They declare the mighty works of Jesus Christ confirmed by the power of the Holy Spirit. When you read the testimonials, keep in mind that although they may not talk about your exact addiction, the biblical principles and victories won can be applied to any addiction — even your addiction! Remember, too, that you have your own story to tell, and your story is going to change in dramatic and surprising ways. It will become more and more wonderful as time goes on, because God says "I know the plans I have for you, plans to prosper you and not to harm you, plans to give you hope and a future" (Jeremiah 29:11, NIV).

Spaced throughout the text are the Scriptures applicable to your walk into freedom. It is so important to read those, meditate on them, speak them, and apply them to your situation in life! There are also prayers written to serve as examples for you if you are not sure how to pray. The sidebars of encouragement and the bulleted lists visually highlight vital information, and I also share some special announcements with insights I know God gave me as I walked my way through this freedom process. I also hope you will find the FAQs and Liberty Tool Kit in the final chapter particularly helpful in adding clarity and ensuring you have applied the freedom principles. Finally, I provide a few appendices at the back for your benefit. They include proclamation cards that you can tear out and carry with you, each Scripture used in the text so that you have all the Scriptures at hand in one place, and a bibliography. My prayer is that the tools I have provided will speed you on your way to a victorious, joy-filled freedom.

What I do not want this book to become is a science or method unto itself. Turning it into a legalistic process won't cut it. It is God's power and presence that does the work, and that is available for everyone. It is about each individual having the truths of our Lord Jesus and His ways revealed to his or her heart and having the faith to believe the truths and see their results. I explain faith simply as "God-Confidence." In other words, there is no doubt that God can and will do what He promised to do for you in His Word. Remember this: God is your sponsor. If He said it—He will back it. So agree with God and believe Him.

I do not profess to know it all regarding this area of freedom from addictions and standing in liberty. As each year goes by, I learn more and more as the Holy Spirit teaches me and reveals more of God's truths to me. So it will be with you. Journey on with the Holy Spirit, and may the Lord God Almighty inspire the truth in your hearts and keep you in all your ways.

PART
1

**Foundations for a
Lifetime of Freedom**

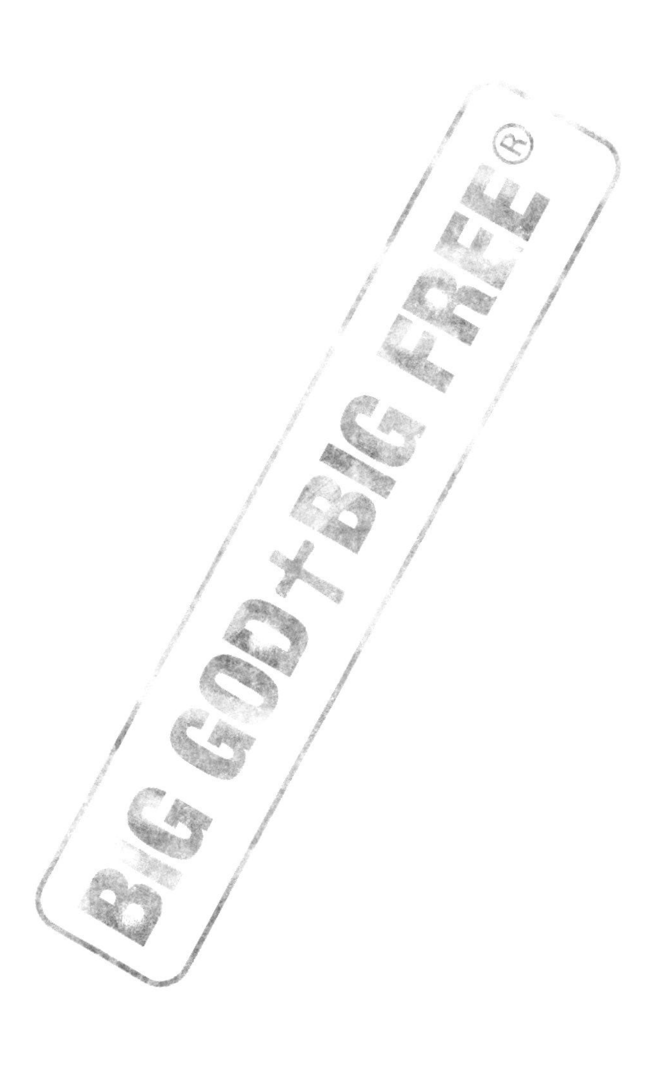

BIG GOD † BIG FREE ®

1
WHO AM I?
Understanding Your Maker's Design

Sally's Story

My life history spans a long trail of abandonment, rejection and emotional abuse. I turned to substances for dulling the pain of my past. I was delivered from alcohol, yet the deception remained that smoking was a less harmful option and a practical defense between me and having that first drink. Later I realized that I had kept the door open to the enemy's influence in my life through accepting these lies. I went to great lengths to hide my smoking from others and to deny my growing dependency on it. I tried to stop many times—to no avail—because my efforts weren't based on what Jesus Christ did for me. They were just different formulas applied in my own strength. Then God showed me the truth: the validity of my need for comfort; the deception I walked in apart from Him to fill that void; and His desire to heal me—right needs / wrong way. When I turned to Him, He not only set me free from cigarettes, but now when I go to Him with my fear, hurt, confusion or stress, He also teaches me how to apply His wisdom so I can walk in victory in those areas that once triggered me to use. I didn't expect the abundance of freedom I am experiencing as He continues to expose the enemy's outrageous lies and perceptual distortions that kept me in physical and emotional bondage. NO butts about it—Go to Him and He will not only snuff out the bondage, He will eradicate the core issues behind it!

We all need a solid foundation on which we can make a stand and claim our freedom. By taking a look at who we are and Whose we are; we can cement in our hearts that solid foundation to build on. Various worldviews and wrong perspectives are unintentionally—and sometimes intentionally—taught to us, but they can provide only a shaky foundation at best. Let's look at God's Truth, starting with who we are

You are the creation of God. Like an author signs a work of art, God signed you! You are a "Designer Original" with God's signature all over you. Isabel Allum brought this point home for me when I heard her Kingdom Identity teaching: "Your parents conceived you, however, God created you." There is a big difference. God knew you before the foundations of the world were formed. He knit you together in your mother's womb, and He loves you and wants you to be His child. (See Psalm 139:1–18.) As I mentioned, all Scriptures I refer to are reproduced in an appendix at the back, "Biblical References," for your benefit.

A CHILD OF GOD

You are a child of God. According to Galatians 4:4–5, "When the time had fully come, God sent His son [Jesus], born of a woman, born under law, to redeem those under the law, that we might receive the full rights of sons [and daughters]" (NIV). As you can see, Jesus made it possible for us to become children of God with full rights to all that God the Father has promised. When you accept Jesus as Lord and Savior and become a child of God, you receive full rights, eternal life, freedom and no condemnation: "For God so loved the world that He gave His only begotten Son, that whoever believes in Him should not perish but have everlasting life. For God did not send His son into the world to condemn the world, but that the world through Him might be saved " (John 3:16–17, NKJV).

In other words, as the great evangelist Smith Wigglesworth put it, Christ showed up to get rid of sin and reconcile us to our Heavenly Father. The most important decision you will ever make in life is turning from your own ways and accepting Jesus as Lord and Savior. When you do this, your name is written in the Lamb's Book of Life and your eternity is sealed. I want to take a minute to share an insight that God gave me:

> *Close your eyes, and I want you to remember a time when you were in a stadium or place where the crowds were going absolutely wild with cheering and shouting. Can you recall what you saw? Can you hear the roar? Good. Now I want you to amplify that by 1 million times. What do you think it would sound like and be like? Well, that doesn't even come close to what all of heaven sounded like when you chose Jesus as Lord and Savior. For the Bible says that all of heaven rejoices—we are talking one big celebration over you!*

We will expand a little further on the level of love the Father has for you, His child, in chapter 2, "Whose Am I?" For now, notice that when there is love, there is no condemnation. God is love, so God never condemns you. Only the enemy does that, satan or the devil, who is called in Scripture the accuser of the brethren (see Revelation 12:10). Romans 8:1–2 indicates, "Therefore, there is now no condemnation for those who are in Christ Jesus, because through Christ Jesus the law of the Spirit of life *set me free* from the law of sin and death" (NIV, italics added). Oh how God loves each one of us, giving us the right to absolute freedom.

WHICH PART OF YOU IS IN CONTROL?

You are made up of three parts, your body (flesh), your soul (mind, will and emotions) and your spirit. By understanding these three parts, you can begin to discern which area of yourself is in control and which one is speaking to you. Note that when you make Jesus your Lord and Savior, you get a new Spirit, God's Spirit, on the inside of you (see Romans 8:11). However, your body and soul did not become new. Your mind, for example, can still come up with some wild and strange thoughts. You might inwardly criticize someone: *Isn't that an ugly shirt that person is wearing?* You may think this while you're being perfectly friendly on the outside. Or you may rationalize with yourself, *Why don't I just do this? No one will see me. They'll never know*…But you can transform your mind over time with the Truth of the Word of God: "Do not conform any longer to the pattern of this world, but be transformed by the renewing of your mind. Then you will be able to test and approve what God's will is—His good, pleasing and perfect will" (Romans 12:2, NIV).

Then there's your body, the flesh. You may be saying, *Wait a minute; you say that my flesh talks to me? Are you some kind of nut?* Nope—it's your flesh that will always be the crazy one. Think about it. Your body tells you when it wants a cigarette, it tells you when it's hungry, it tells you when it's tired or something hurts. That is how it talks to you. Historically, your flesh has been in control. It has told you when to have a cigarette, or maybe when to overeat or when to drink or when to indulge in any number of other addictions. It is constantly craving and constantly trying to tell you what to do. The apostle Paul experienced this with his flesh, too. He said, "With my mind I myself serve the law of God, but with the flesh the law of sin" (Romans 7:25, NKJV).

Part of your struggle and mine with addictions and other difficult areas is that we sometimes let the wrong part of us have authority over the other parts. What we are going to do throughout our process here is change the order of authority among our three parts. You go forward by increasing the might of your spirit to subdue your flesh and by renewing your mind with God's Word. Your flesh and your soul(mind, will, and emotions) may not want to be subdued, but they have to be in order to make progress. The Spirit of God will help you get your parts in order!

Because God's Spirit came to live on the inside of you when you made Him Lord and Savior, your body is now the temple of God. First Corinthians 3:16 tells us, "Don't you know that you yourselves are God's temple and that God's Spirit lives in you?" (NIV). Therefore, if God lives in you, you'll want to examine yourself, clean and purify yourself as He is pure. The Bible says, "And everyone who has this hope in Him [Jesus] purifies himself, just as He is pure" (1 John 3:3, NKJV).

Holiness and purity are simply being absolutely clean and without compromise, in line with God's ways. Who doesn't want that? A place of total freedom, where nothing from the enemy influences or affects you. God wants us to examine ourselves so He doesn't have to. Believe me; it is a lot easier to examine ourselves than to be examined later by God. Like King David, after he committed adultery and then realized it was wrong, we need to repent of sin (turn from practicing it anymore) and ask God to forgive us and make in us a clean and pure heart. The blood of Jesus can clean anything.

OVERCOMING LIFE'S BUMPS, HUMPS AND ENEMY ATTACHMENTS

Each person's journey through life will include both peaks and valleys. Part of our role is to discipline ourselves just as an athlete goes through the discipline of training for a big event or race. How do we do this? We bring our bodies and souls into subjection under our spirit. Look what the apostle Paul said about this in 1 Corinthians 9:24–27 (NIV):

> *Do you not know that in a race all the runners run, but only one gets the prize? Run in such a way as to get the prize. Everyone who competes in the games goes into strict training. They do it to get a crown that will not last; but we do it to get a crown that will last forever. Therefore . . . I beat my body and make it my slave so that after I have preached to others, I myself will not be disqualified for the prize.*

So how should we continue our life journey? By disciplining ourselves to run to win. Hebrews 12:1–2 adds, "Let us throw off everything that hinders and the sin that so easily entangles, and let us run with perseverance the race marked out for us. Let us fix our eyes on Jesus, the author and perfecter of our faith . . ." (NIV). The crown of life is for the overcomer (see James 1:12 and Revelation 2:10–11), so expect life to have its twists and turns. When I read Psalm 23:4, I always wish it would say "Yea, though I pass *over* the valley of the shadow of death" instead of "Yea, though I walk *through* it." But I know that we will walk through some tough times in life, and that same verse also says <u>God will be with us</u> to comfort us in those times. In later chapters, we will examine some more specific ways and means of overcoming in tough times. Read on and race on—your destiny and your crown await you!

TEST YOURSELF—WHO ARE YOU?

- ☐ Are you God's or the Devil's?
- ☐ Are you a child of the Most High God?
- ☐ Is Jesus Christ your Lord and Savior?
- ☐ Are you who the heavenly Father says you are or who the world says you are?
- ☐ Are you who the heavenly Father says you are or who your family says you are?
- ☐ Are you who the heavenly Father says you are or who your coworkers, neighbors, friends and community say you are?
- ☐ Are you who you were (your past) or who the Heavenly Father says you are?

2
WHOSE AM I?
Amazing Truths About Your Maker

> ***Pastor D's Story:*** *Before I got saved I was a smoker. When I got born again, my spirit got saved and made new but my flesh didn't. So, here I was with a new spirit and I didn't want to keep smoking cigarettes anymore. I gave it up, but my flesh screamed at me the next day, saying "I want a Winston cigarette now!"*
>
> *I said, "No, you are not getting one."*
>
> *It screamed again, "I want a Winston now!"*
>
> *I said, "No!"*
>
> *This went on several times, and then my body said, "Okay, how about a Marlboro then?"*
>
> *I said, "No!" My flesh tried just about every brand of cigarette, and I kept saying, "No!" My flesh spoke to me, and I spoke back to it in the name of Jesus. My spirit won!*

Oftentimes, we tend to view our relationships with others and view who others are through our own lenses and experiences. Sometimes this is good and sometimes it is not, because sometimes it can give us a distorted or incomplete view of how things really are. In particular, I find myself and many others viewing God the Father and our relationship with Him through the lenses of how we viewed our earthly fathers. Even if your earthly father is a good man, he is human and cannot begin to represent who God the Father really is. And if we have had fathers who misused or abused us in their own weaknesses and sin, that makes it very difficult to even imagine how good our heavenly Father is and that He loves us. Many times our earthly fathers don't know how to express their love. Sometimes they physically abandon us, are distant, or pull away from us in other ways, which can taint our view of how much our heavenly Father loves us. In this section, let's take a closer look at Whose we are—at the amazing truth about who God the Father really is and what He thinks about you His child.

GOD IS A TRIUNE GOD

God is three in one: God the Father (referred to as the Father from here on), God the Son (who is Jesus Christ) and God the Spirit (who is the Holy Spirit). We must remember that they are truly three in one. In other words, there is no dysfunction or disagreement between them. There is also no jealousy, so if you like Jesus, you like the Father and the Holy Spirit, too.

Often, we can believe that Jesus loves us, but we are not so sure about God the Father. I mean, He is God, Omni-everything! That's an ominous thought to some of us, but a simple truth was revealed to me in John 14:7. Jesus says in effect, "If you know me, you know the Father." They are the same, they are one! God the Father loves you, just as Jesus loves you. How awesome is that! "How great is the love the Father has lavished on us, that we should be called children of God! And that is what we are!" says 1 John 3:1 (NIV). This is amazing—the Father *lavishes* His love on us. We are not talking a few drops here or there, on some days but not other days. It is every day, in unfathomable amounts, *lavished* on us. Here's an analogy I like that demonstrates the term *lavish*:

I like peanut butter and jelly sandwiches (PBJs). Does anyone else? The way I can image what the word lavish means is by thinking about how I put my peanut butter on my PBJ. It is about two inches thick and covers every part of the bread possible, plus it hangs over the sides! In a word, I lavish the peanut butter on my PBJ.

This is a simple analogy, but how much more lavish is the truth about how God loves us. His love is unconditional, extravagant, boundless and fathomless. So receive it. Be lavished upon with God's love, starting today!

GOD IS A GOD OF COVENANT

God has given us His written Word, and He watches over it to perform it (see Jeremiah 1:12). According to John 1:1, Jesus is the Word: "In the beginning was the Word, and the Word was with God, and the Word was God" (NIV)

Many think, *So what's the big deal about the Word?* For starters, the Word of God is living. It is powerful—more powerful than a two-edged sword. Hebrews 4:12 says so: "For the word of God is living and powerful, and sharper than any two-edged sword, piercing even to the division of soul and spirit, and of joints and marrow, and is a discerner of the thoughts and intents of the heart" (NKJV). God spoke, and His Word created the earth and all that is in it. The power of God is unleashed when He speaks, and His Word never goes out without accomplishing His purposes. God is a God of covenant. If He said something, He will do it! No questions asked, because there is no variableness or changing in Him. According to 2 Corinthians 1:20, all of God's promises are yes, <u>in Christ</u> and through Him Amen! The Bible is full of God's promises, and He is the same yesterday, today and tomorrow. He will be faithful to perform His Word.

I like the what Hebrews 10:23 says: "Let's keep a firm grip on the promises that keep us going. He always keeps his word" (MESSAGE). This means that we have to move our focus from our problems or circumstances onto God's promises. How do we do this? We begin to return God's Word to Him. We find out what He says in His Word about a situation, we proclaim it (believe it in our hearts and speak it out of our mouths), and we receive it. This is faith, "the substance of things hoped for, the evidence of things not seen" (Hebrews 11:1, KJV). Faith isn't a feeling, and faith never looks about doubtfully. Remember when Peter tried to walk on the water to Jesus and then started looking about doubtfully at the wind and waves? Peter started to sink because he got his eyes off of Jesus and onto his situation (see Matthew 14:25–31). Better to keep your eyes on your Savior and His Truth, never mind the circumstances.

The gospel of Jesus is always Good News. According to Hebrews 12:2, Jesus is the Author and the Finisher of our faith. He authored it, He brought all the good things into being, and He finished it. He finished it, as He Himself proclaimed on the cross: "'It is finished.' With that, He bowed His head and gave up His spirit" (John 19:30, NIV). Therefore, there is nothing left for us to do to "earn" salvation, healing or freedom—it has been done, past tense. Jesus destroyed the works of the enemy (see 1 John 3:8), reconciled us to God and made available all of God's promises—what a relief! Jesus started it and finished it. All we need to do is get in line with God's will, believe, stay in line with God's will, and receive that which He bought for us.

The Holy Spirit confirms the Word of God. When we repent, believe and receive, the Holy Spirit confirms it all. The Holy Spirit is our comforter, our teacher, our counselor, the anointing power of God that destroys the yoke of sin and lifts burdens. All that Jesus did on earth, which was the will of the Father, was done through the Holy Spirit's anointing. When you believed and asked Jesus to be your Lord and Savior, the Holy Spirit confirmed this by coming to live on the inside of you. The Holy Spirit performs the Word and confirms it. The very same Holy Spirit Who raised Jesus from the dead wants to confirm life, liberty and health to you today. Invite Him in to stay.

GOD'S FREE GIFTS

Who isn't into free gifts? God the Father has arranged and provided so many free gifts for us through the work of Jesus Christ. We must get it straight, though—the first thing we need to know is that we have nothing to do with providing these things. They are gifts. We cannot buy, we cannot earn, and we cannot sell God's gifts. "Every good and perfect gift is from above, coming down from the Father of heavenly lights, who does not change like shifting shadows" (James 1:17, NIV). If something isn't good, it isn't from God. Remember, He doesn't change. He gives only good gifts.

The second thing we need to know is that not only is Jesus the Word, but He is also, as we said, the Author and the Finisher of our faith in that Word. He authored it and finished it - just receive it! How awesome, Jesus paid the Price! Jesus Paid the Price! Jesus Paid the Price! The Bible says Jesus came that we might have life and have it abundantly (see John 10:10).

What does *abundantly* mean and what are those good gifts? Look sometime at Isaiah chapters 58 and 61 as well as what Jesus did while He was here on Earth. Jesus was the will of the Father in action. He did only the Father's will and represents what God wants for you.

Here are just a few of the gifts of God's abundant life:

- ☐ Eternal life
- ☐ Good tidings
- ☐ Binding up of a broken heart
- ☐ Liberty to the captives and the oppressed
- ☐ Joy and gladness
- ☐ Peace that passes all understanding
- ☐ Beauty for ashes
- ☐ Oil of Joy for mourning
- ☐ Garment of praise for the spirit of heaviness
- ☐ Healing of all diseases
- ☐ Prosperity and favor
- ☐ Deliverance from enemy influence and torment
- ☐ Forgiveness of sins

- ☐ Repair of the breach
- ☐ Restoration of the paths
- ☐ Mercy and grace
- ☐ Faith, hope and love
- ☐ The fruits of the Spirit

The list could go on and on. What a great exchange for us to take part in. But why the free gifts? So that He might be glorified. Check it out in His Word. God is omnipotent and omnipresent—He is a _Big God!_ He is bigger than any problem or hang-up we have. Let Him be God and remove them today. Let Him be God and give you something better.

Pick up your Bible and repeat after me:"This is my Bible. I can have what it says I can have. It is the Truth of God."

GOD IS A GOD OF PURPOSE

God has a specific purpose for you and for me. As we saw earlier, He intricately made you exactly the way He wanted you, a unique design for this time and for this place. He wrote on your heart desires that are in line with His desires, and He will bring you great joy as you fulfill them. Spend time with Him and these desires will bubble up.There is no striving in this purpose, just rest. Second Timothy 2:9 tells us God "has saved us and called us to a holy life—not because of anything we have done but because of his own purpose and grace. This grace was given us in Christ Jesus before the beginning of time" (NIV). Our identity is in God and His love, nothing else.

It is clear that God has a great purpose for you, which is why the enemy tries so hard to get you off track and powerless. All are called but few respond, so today choose to run your race that God has set before you, "being confident of this, that he who began a good work in you will carry it to completion until the day of Christ Jesus" (Philippians 1:6, NIV). His work in you only stops when Jesus returns. It is never too late, and you are never too far gone! No matter where you are, where you have been or where you think you are headed, as Romans 8:39 says, nothing can separate you from the Love of God.

God always loves you, and you cannot change that. He may not like what you are *doing*, but He always loves *you* and wants *you* to be His child. God has a great purpose for you—choose His way and be mighty in spirit and full of His power. Remember:

- ☐ Don't exchange God's plans for fear or a feeling.
- ☐ Don't exchange God's plans for what others think it should be.
- ☐ Don't exchange God's plans for any reason. His plans are the best plans for your good life.

You have a call to fulfill—be on your way!

WHOSE YOU ARE NOT—THE DEVIL AND YOUR OTHER FOES

Sometimes we like to live in a fantasy land and believe that we do not have enemies. But God's Word warns very clearly that we should not be ignorant or be deceived. In fact, we have three major categories of enemies: the devil and his forces, the world system, and our own flesh. It is difficult to win any battle if we don't understand who our enemies are and what their game is. Like a good military strategist, let's take a look at these three enemies and how they make war against us.

The devil and his forces. The devil is the fallen angel Lucifer, who when he fell took a third of God's angels with him. These fallen angels now comprise his demonic forces. Ephesians 6:12 instructs us: "For our struggle is not against flesh and blood [other people], but against the rulers, against the authorities, against the powers of this dark world and against the spiritual forces of evil in the heavenly realms" (NIV). It is not people we wrestle against, but rather the enemy forces that often influence people to play out their game. We must always remember it is not the person but rather the enemy force behind the person that is the source of our trouble.

The world system. The world and its ways are also our enemy. 1 John 2:15–17 (NIV).warns,

> *Do not love the world or anything in the world. If anyone loves the world, the love of the Father is not in him. For everything in the world—the cravings of sinful man, the lust of his eyes and the boasting of what he has and does—comes not from the Father but from the world. The world and its desires pass away, but the man who does the will of God lives forever.*

The things of the world will never satisfy and will require you to keep going back or going for more. Remember, the devil is the god with a little "g" of this world, according to Scripture and we as believers are to be in the world, but not of it. You can only serve one master and where your treasure is, there your heart is also.

Our crazy flesh. Our flesh is also our enemy. Galatians 5:16–17 tells us to walk in the spirit so we do not fulfill the lust of the flesh because "the flesh lusts against the Spirit, and the Spirit against the flesh; and these are contrary to one another; so that you do not do the things that you wish" (NKJV). What does the work of the flesh life look like? Galatians 5 goes on to tell us: idolatry, adultery, fornication, uncleanness, lewdness, revelries, witchcraft, sorcery, hatred, wrath, strife, gossip, jealousies, heresies, outbursts of wrath, murder, drunkenness, envying, and other such things. And it warns that those who do such things shall not inherit the kingdom of God (verses 19–21). We must live in the spirit and crucify our flesh and its desires.

THE ENEMIES' STRATEGY AND GAMES

Now that we have a clear idea of who our enemies are, let's take a look at their strategy and games. This is not meant to be an exhaustive list, but rather highlights some of their major tactics. We know that the intent of any of our enemies is to harm us, not do us good. They plot evil against us and those around us.

The devil and his forces. The outcome the devil and his forces desire is clear in John 10:10, which states that the devil comes to steal, to kill and to destroy us. That's just the opposite of Jesus, who came that we might have life and life abundantly. If you are being robbed inside or out, parts of your life are dying, or you feel decimated, you know the enemy is attacking. We know his intent is to kill, steal or destroy, so if you see any of these three in your situation, you know who is behind it.

The devil is also the father of all lies. One of his greatest strategies is to bend the truth (sometimes slightly and sometimes greatly) and see if he can get you to agree to it and go with it. John 8:44 says of those who go his way, "You belong to your father, the devil, and you want to carry out your father's desire. He was a murderer from the beginning, not holding to the truth, for there is no truth in him. When he lies, he speaks his native language, for he is a liar and the father of lies" (NIV). That is why we must test all things, including our words and actions and also what others do and say, against the Word of God, which is absolute truth. If it doesn't line up, and I mean completely, it is not of God but rather of the devil. God is a full-truth, not a half-truth, God.

The world system. The world and the things of this world try to distract us from God—all those things that so many of us chase after and try to obtain. It is not that the things of this world are all bad; they are not. The problem arises when they control you and drive you. It is the love of it that is the determining factor. A man cannot have two masters, God and money, for he will love the one and hate the other, says Scripture (see Matthew 6:24). You either love the world or you love God. What you love is the determining factor in what influences your life and whether you win your battles. Take a lesson from wise King Solomon, who exceeded in all things (riches, wisdom) beyond even the richest man today. Solomon said in Ecclesiastes 1:14 that the things of this world are all vanity and vexation of spirit. In other words, they are meaningless and frustrating, like chasing after the wind. I ask myself the following questions often, and the answers are always enlightening:

☐ Where do I spend my time and effort, with whom, and for what?

☐ Am I driven by the distractions of the world, or am I led by the Spirit?

Now that you have a view of your enemies and their games, remember, "Greater is He that is in you, than he that is in the world" (1 John 4:4, KJV). You are a conqueror, an overcomer, an heir of God Almighty, with full authority and the right to be free from the bondage the enemy tries to get you into and tie you up with. Don't play his game, don't fall for the lies, and don't get distracted. The enemy forces can only gain influencing control of that which is yielded to them. If you don't yield it, they can have no part in it, because as a child of God, you are under God's protection. Keep your eyes on Jesus and you will be alright. *The game is already won!* Take up your shield of faith and take a victory lap!

Our crazy flesh. The primary strategy of our flesh is to reverse the authority order. It is a power struggle between our flesh and our spirit (see Romans 7:19). When you accept Jesus as Lord and Savior, you get a new spirit on the inside of you and you become a child of God. However, your flesh does not get changed in this process. It still wants all those crazy things it wanted before (like ten pieces of pizza instead of two or to cuss and swear). If the flesh can make you believe that you cannot subdue it or control it with your spirit, it wins. Proverbs 24:28 tells us, "Like a city whose walls are broken down is a man who lacks self-control" (NIV). Another way you could phrase that is "a man who is under flesh control."

The realm of the flesh is where the devil tries to entice and seduce you into fulfilling those thoughts and imaginations he plants in your head. Your head (mind) is the battleground. It is connected to your body, and the enemy knows it. He tries to get them working together to desire and go after wrong things and open the door to him. The good news though, is "that which is born of the Spirit is spirit" (John 3:6, NIV)—we can choose to walk in the Spirit versus walking in the flesh. We can cast down vain (useless) imaginations and tell them to go in Jesus' name.

As Jesse Duplantis would say, "Grab your flesh by the ear, and command it to line up with God and stay in its cage, in Jesus' name."

3
GOD'S ROOTS OF RIGHTEOUSNESS
What is Behind This Addiction?

MICHELLE'S STORY: I was prone to outbursts of anger and I smoked for over 20 years – though no one knew it. I hid it well. Cigarettes were my friend and my comfort and I was their slave. I danced with anger. I didn't want to admit it but I had a few heart wounds. My earthly father (who is a great man but also human) seemed to express his love in minimal quantities. He was busy starting and running his own business, and because of his work-orientated focus I thought the basis for receiving more of his love and attention was to perform and achieve. I became a performance junkie with a walled up heart—telling myself the habits didn't matter. The great ending to this story is that I came into the Truth – that God the Father loves me unconditionally and I could get free. I repented of my wrongful ways, my poor choices, and my reaching to other people and things instead of God. I forgave my father, repented of dishonoring him, and I got free! WOW — Thank you Jesus, for setting me at liberty.

JAMES'S STORY: I was an alcoholic and smoked for over 53 years. In fact, my mother smoked while I was in her womb. I don't blame her, though, for my habit. I made the choice to start and to keep smoking. I was delivered of alcoholism and many other addictions, but I didn't seem to be able to let go of the smoking. Praise God, I finally repented of my rebellion and did let it go! I stand delivered—the wounds behind my addictions were healed with the love of God. Praise the name of the Lord. Nothing is too big for Him!

As I stated in the Introduction, the difference with the approach you will find in these pages is that it deals with the root behind your addiction. Personally, I tried over and over again to quit my addiction, smoking. I had never asked God, though, to show me what was behind the addiction, driving me to become addicted in the first place. I needed God's help in discovering and dealing with the root. I call what was at the root of it all a wound, because that's exactly what it is behind any addictive behavior—a heart wound. Back then I didn't realize that the hurts in my heart were the driving force behind my addiction and what I had become.

We live our lives in a fallen world system, which means you and I are going to receive damage and get wounded in this life by fallen mankind and lurking enemies. Your wound or wounds can come from many places; you may know when and where you got them, or you may not know. Let's go a little deeper into these wounds of the heart. As we do, remember the ones I mention are not an all encompassing list. There may be many other wounds or reasons behind your addictions, but the good news is that God can take care of them <u>all</u> through the blood of Jesus. He heals and restores—Scripture first says He came to "bind up the brokenhearted." He came to proclaim freedom for the captives and release from darkness for the prisoners. If you thought you would always be a prisoner to your addiction, held captive by its power over you, He has news for you! He came for this very reason: so that you might be free!

Part of what you will do later in the ministry section is ask God to reveal to you the specific root, and wounds, behind your addiction. Then you will ask Him to remove the roots and replace it with the His love and new roots of righteousness. If you don't get the roots removed, you might have a shot at overcoming your present addiction anyway, but that root is going to grow back just like a vine. If you break or cut a vine but don't remove the root, it will be there again next year, maybe in a different shape and size, but it will keep growing. In other words, other addictions may then take the place of the one you are struggling with now. Better to remove the source this time around!

Often, a primary root of addictions is delivered and deposited in our hearts through some form of being or feeling unloved, like abuse, rejection, divorce, abandonment and so forth. I believe that because God is Love, the enemy ferociously tries to attack and wound us in our love for God, ourselves or others. Singer Tina Turner had it all wrong asking "What's love got to do with it?" Love has *everything* to do with us. Take a look at what the New Testament focuses on. God says all the way through that love is what it is all about—loving Him, loving ourselves and loving others. One time when I asked God what life is all about, He gave me this song:

What's It All About
It's all about Loving God
It's all about Loving Others
No matter the Cost.

It's all about Loving God
It's all about Loving Others
No Matter the Cost.

It's all about being in His presence
And taking a drink of His living water,
Then going after the Hurt and the Lost.

It's all about Loving God
It's all about Loving Others
No Matter the Cost.

Stephen Covey even talks about how one of the principle cornerstones for humans is to love and be loved. Face it, we want to be celebrated and loved, and that is a good thing. So of course, that is where the enemy attacks the hardest. Let's call such wounds unloving wounds. Once you are wounded, the enemy then plants and attaches roots of rebellion, anger, jealousy and so forth.

HOW UNLOVING WOUNDS HAPPEN

The enemy typically tries to deliver an unloving wound to your heart through the following means:

Abuse. When you don't know something's purpose (in particular God's purpose for it) and you don't have love, you abuse it. Abuse is rampant in our society today. There are four types of abuse—physical, verbal, spiritual and sexual. Often it is through these means that the enemy delivers a major wound. In God's eyes any abuse is wrong and contrary to His love and purpose for you. In ministry sessions, it is typical that within a group, more than 75 percent of the individuals have been abused in some way, often horrifically.

Generational sins and curses. Another method the enemy uses to get to you is through your family. Let's face it, we all have dysfunctional families, the only difference is the magnitude of dysfunction. There is a spiritual law that says the sins and iniquities of the fathers are passed on to the third and fourth generations unless they are broken (see Exodus 34:6–7). So often, when we don't even know where the root came from and why we do the things that we do, a generational sin or curse may need to be broken. Now you see that it could be a great-great-grandfather who sinned and brought the curse, but its consequences affect us, a future generation. Again, Jesus paid the price and in Him, we have the power to break those off our lives and our children's lives.

Oftentimes you also see generations of people who don't know how to love each other. Look at people who don't know how to love their children, and you will often see that they were dealt with in a similar fashion, unloved by their own parents. This is no excuse for their actions, but it often points to the source of their wounds and the roots behind them. You may have heard the phrase "wounded people wound others." This proves very true, whether they do it intentionally or unintentionally.

Disobedience to God's ways. Unloving wounds that damage faith, hope, and love often start as the result of someone's actions, not necessarily your own. The actions were contrary to God's ways (the best ways) and ended up deeply affecting you. For example, abandonment, divorce, sexual immorality, absentee parents, anger, jealousy, separation, bitterness, rejection, betrayal and so forth comprise these wounds. These all open the door to the enemy and allow him to enter and deliver a heart wound, both to those who practice these things and to the those around them who are affected by the actions.

UNWELCOME ATTACHMENTS

Once an initial wound is delivered and the enemy plants the root of an unloving wound in your heart, he then tries to attach as many other hurtful things as possible to it. The primary root deposited into the wound, as you can see from the illustration, is unlovingness, then all of its attachments branch off from it.

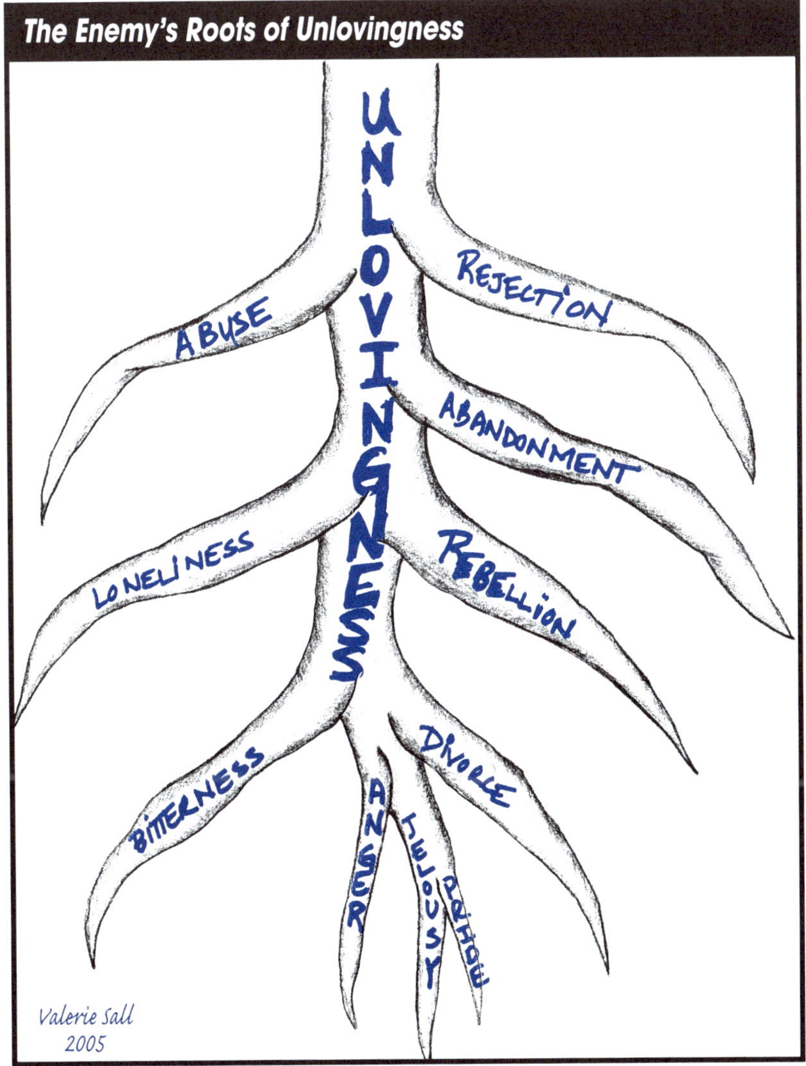

REPLACEMENT ROOTS

The good news is that Jesus paid the price to have all of these roots that were deposited by the enemy, pulled out and replaced with the love of God and roots of righteousness. The illustration shows how the roots of righteousness are love, faith and hope, with all of the fruits of the Spirit attached—peace, joy, gentleness, kindness, mercy, and the rest (see Galatians 5:22–23).

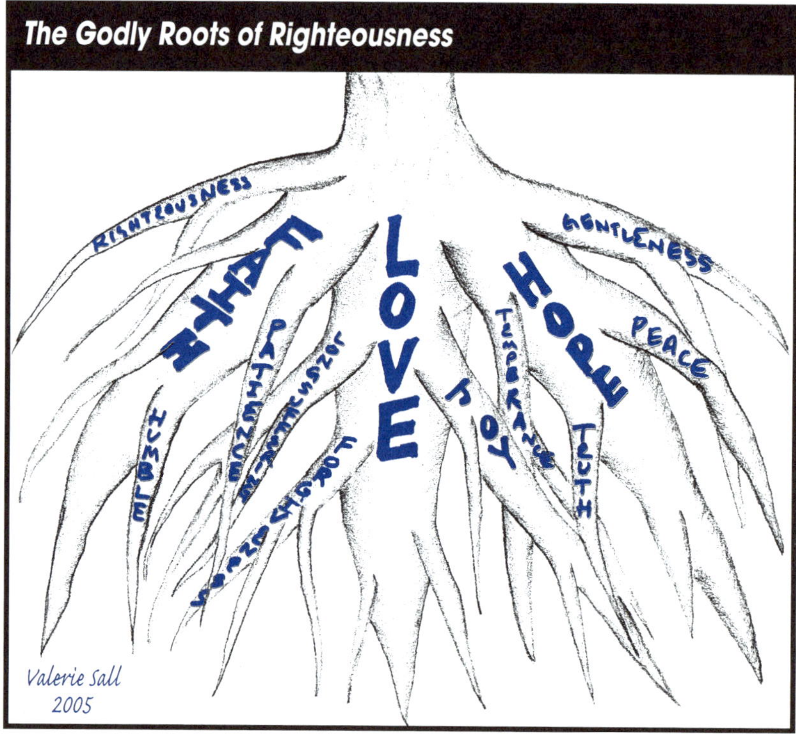

Part of our approach here is asking God to remove the roots the enemy planted and replace them with His love. Got enemy roots? Don't worry - you are in common company and God wants to remove them *all* today! God's love can *always* go deeper than any root of the enemy! This isn't a maybe kind of process; this is complete, 100 percent eradication and replacement—if you want it, it is yours. *For what you give up—He takes and what you hang on to—you keep.*

WHY AM I ADDICTED?

As you can see, the roots of the enemy cause your flesh to rise up over your spirit, and they leave a gaping hole in your heart that needs to be filled. There are two ways to fill this, with the lust of the flesh, which will never completely satisfy and give pleasure only for a season (see Hebrews 11:25), or with God's love, which will satisfy completely. Remember the story of the woman at the well? I heard T. D. Jakes talk about the revelation in that story once. He said something like this:

> *The woman at the well had had five previous husbands and a current circumstance (boyfriend). I mean, this is adultery and uncleanness to the hilt. But what Jesus said to her was, "You are thirsty and until you drink of my living water (Jesus and His love) you will thirst." In other words, you will keep going somewhere to get that love need met again and again and again. Jesus didn't condemn her, rather He said, "Drink from my cup—drink the living water and you won't need that anymore."*

For me, cigarettes were a friend and I enjoyed them, but I kept wanting to quit. I knew they were not good for me, and they influenced me (my body basically demanded a cigarette when I needed one, and they consumed my time and money). Once I recognized that I had a wounded heart, I repented and asked God to remove the enemy's root and the wounds and replace them with His love for me. I asked Him to deliver me and destroy the yoke of addiction. He did, and that's what made the difference—wow, what a difference! The enemy still tried to tempt me back, but to no avail. I was sticking with God and sticking with His real thing—God's Love and God's plans!

WHY CHANGE?

So why are you addicted? Simple: You have a wounded heart that has driven you. Don't be ashamed, everyone does in some way. Life happens to you, and many times it hurts. Those hurts can cause us to do things we don't like and become someone we don't want to be. The good news is you don't have to keep the hurt—you can exchange it. You can change. The choice is yours. Maybe addictions are a friend to you, too, as they were to me. Maybe they make you feel good, maybe they are always there, maybe you think you are cool because of them, maybe they are a form of rebellion or escape. Let them go and get something better—something that lasts forever!

Don't be like Pharaoh who chose to spend one more night with the plague of frogs before he gave in and became obedient to God's command (see Exodus 8:8–10). You can be like that, but it isn't any fun. It is only the enemy trying to keep you down at his level and out of the good things that God has for you. Sin and bondage are a major disruption to God's order and your destiny. God has a wonderful purpose and destiny for you. You will never be able to live it, fulfill it and enjoy it completely until you make the exchange and get free. The accuser, the devil, will always have a foothold on you and hinder your witness and your standard of living. But once Jesus sets you free and plants new roots of love and righteousness in your heart, you will never want to go back to "Egypt" (like the Israelites wanted to) and be a slave to the things that once held you captive!

HOW IS THIS PROCESS DIFFERENT?

This process is different from other ways of dealing with addictions. First, as we just said, it eradicates the root of your addiction and replaces it with something better; God's love. Also, it is God's power in you, working in your spirit. If you were like me and hadn't thought to ask for God's help until now, this process—and your success rate—will be a whole new experience for you! Inside you is God's Spirit, and He's going to increase *your* spiritual might and your will to stand in liberty over what might have been a weakness in the past. Today, we are going to ignite the dynamite power of God. Think of this analogy:

Remember the cartoon where Wile E. Coyote would try to dynamite the Road Runner? He put the pile of dynamite out and fixed a string back to the activator. Like Wile E. had to push down the activator to get the dynamite to blow up, you will need to take some faith steps to activate God's Freedom Power in your life. The Road Runner may never have succumbed to Wile E. Coyote's efforts, but the power of God's Living Word can blow every addiction and bondage in your life to bits!

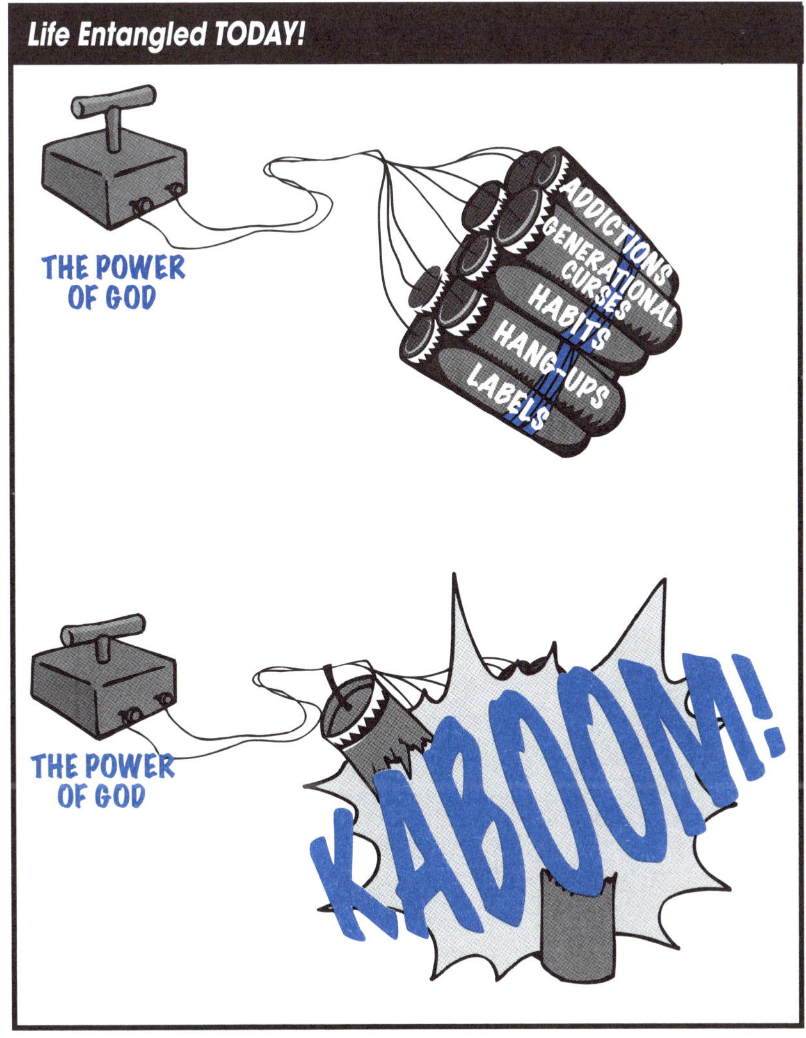

BIG GOD†BIG FREE®

PART
2

Removal and Replacement Principles

or

Addiction Out, Freedom In!

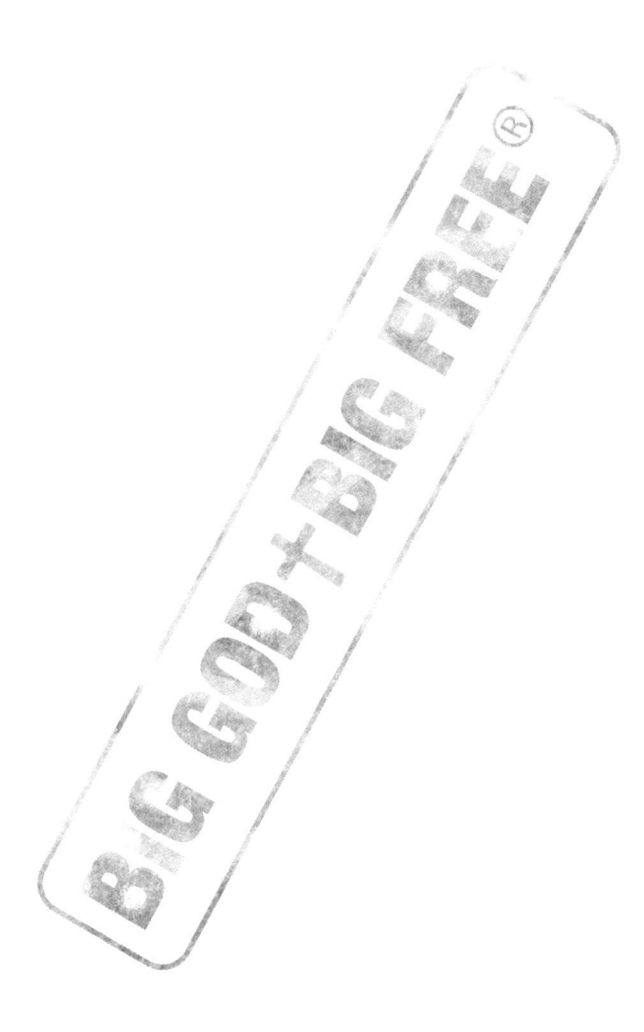
BIG GOD † BIG FREE ®

4
OUT WITH THE OLD
AND IN WITH THE NEW!
The Eradication and Replacement Approach

TOM'S STORY: I want to share a story of how I was delivered of smoking marijuana. I kept falling into the smoking scene, until God came to me one night while I was hanging out with a group of drug users. So here I was, in the middle of this group, and the presence of God hit me, warning me that if I continued on the path, I was facing certain destruction and certain death. I said "I need to get free" and the next morning sought help. My wife and I found the closest church. I repented and asked God to free me. I then found a church where the pastor continued to teach me about God, Jesus and the Holy Spirit and got healed. I now have a beautiful daughter and a family of my own. With God in my life, I continue to grow stronger every day. My life is better than it ever was before. Thank You, Lord, for setting me free.

The approach of eradication and replacement, which simply put means out with the old ways and in with the new, is built upon the things we have covered so far and the following building blocks: Jesus paid the price, the Holy Spirit's anointing destroys the yoke of bondage, it is the Living Word, and standing fast, which includes the concepts of confession and belief, repentance and renunciation, and grace and forgiveness. Let's take a little bit deeper look into each of these to ensure we have a clear and simple understanding.

JESUS PAID THE PRICE

Jesus paid the price with His precious blood so that we could be totally free and reconciled to God the Father. Jesus paid the price with His incorruptible life so the following promise He bought for us is incorruptible as well: "Therefore, there is now no condemnation for those who are in Christ Jesus, because through Christ Jesus the law of the Spirit of life *set me free* from the law of sin and death"(Romans 8:1–2, NIV, italics added). Jesus bought you freedom. John 8:36 says, "So if the Son [Jesus] sets you free, you will be free indeed."

We can be free because Jesus paid the price and is offering us the gift of freedom and restoration. Take it. "For we know that our old self was crucified with Him so that the body of sin might be rendered powerless, that we should no longer be slaves to sin," says Romans 6:6 (NIV). Jesus paid the ultimate price, so don't allow the price He paid to be for nothing. Your freedom has already been bought.

TAKE IT, TAKE IT, TAKE IT!
JESUS PAID THE PRICE!
HE SHED HIS PRECIOUS BLOOD!
HE WANTS TO COVER YOU IN HIS LOVE!
OH WHAT A PRICE HE PAID!
TAKE IT, TAKE IT, TAKE IT!
IT'S FREEDOM AND IT'S FREE!
IT'S FREE TO YOU AND IT'S FREE TO ME!

THE HOLY SPIRIT'S ANOINTING
DESTROYS THE YOKE OF BONDAGE

The Holy Spirit is part of the Triune God. He is the one who confirms the Word and the promises of God through powerful signs and wonders. If you look back through your Bible, you will see that while Jesus was on the earth, all that He did was the will of the Father and He did it under the anointing of the Holy Spirit. When the Holy Spirit was upon Him, He performed miracles, healings, and deliverances, and even raised the dead. That same Holy Spirit is alive and well today. Even better, now that Jesus has paid the price, the Holy Spirit lives inside of us instead of upon us. He is waiting to perform and confirm the Word of the Lord. How powerful is that anointing—it is yoke destroying and burden lifting (see Isaiah 10:27). It is the fulfillment of God's Word, which shatters the rock or the stony parts of our hearts, then gives us hearts of flesh that can receive the love of God. (see Ezekiel 11:19). One of my mentors, Reverend Alex Chavez, has a great analogy of this that he uses:

> *Pick up a stone; if you tried to pour water into that stone, it wouldn't receive it. It would hit the stone and spray off the sides. Now if that stone was changed and made soft, it could receive what you are trying to pour into it. God wants you to receive His love and His living water, by giving you a better and new heart.*

We can do nothing without the Blood of Jesus and the Holy Spirit—they do all the work. Never be deceived—it is not any person who does the work, no matter where you are or who is praying with you or for you. It is all God's work and ministry.

LIVING WORD

The Word of God is Living Word. It brings life to those who hear it and believe it. It is *alive*—powerful and effectual—dividing joints, discerning thoughts and hearts—it is life changing (see Hebrews 4:12). According to John 6:63, "The Spirit gives life; the flesh counts for nothing. The words I have spoken to you are spirit and they are life" (NIV).

LIVING WORD, LIVING WORD!
DRINK IT IN, DRINK IT IN!
THE POWER IS IN THE WORD OF GOD.
(JESUS WAS THE WORD IN FLESH)
IT IS LIVING WORD, IT IS LIVING WORD.
IT WILL CHANGE YOU IF YOU CONSUME IT AND LET IT.

In Mark 13:31, Jesus also tells us "Heaven and earth will pass away, but my words will never pass away" (NIV). Not only is it Living Word, it is Eternal Word. Good today, good tomorrow, good next year. This means everything in His Word is for today—healing, restoration, deliverance and salvation. Many people are deceived by the enemy's lies that these things were only for biblical times, but when you read the Word, it is clear that they are for <u>now</u> and forever and that God has not changed. Believe and take it—it is Good News!

STANDING FAST

How does one stand fast? An analogy I like to use is if a mighty wind comes up and you are outside with nowhere to go for shelter, you are going to stand fast. You will try to put your feet into something, you will try to hang on to something, you will try to make yourself heavy somehow like an anchor, you will turn your back to the wind so it doesn't hit your face, and you will cry out for help. You will do whatever you can with whatever you have to make it through the storm.

It takes the same thing to stand fast against eradicated addictions. Once Jesus sets you free, you are forever free, yet you still need to stand fast in your liberty; for the enemy will try to coax you away from that freedom and seduce you back into the addiction. The devil is upset he lost you and wants you back. Don't let him entangle you again!

Remember the parable of the sower and the seeds? The enemy wants to steal your seed—your freedom—while it is freshly planted, because the deeper the good roots of God's liberty go and the more you taste freedom, the less chance he has of getting you to give it up.

Confess and Believe. At the end of the day, you need confidence in order to stand fast. It is all about confidence, and it must be "God-confidence," not self-confidence. God-confidence is Faith. It means that you confess and believe God will do what He said He would. *He will* deliver you and set you free, *He will* heal you, *He will* protect you, *He will* meet you in your weakness, *He will* provide a way out when you are tempted, *He will never* leave you nor forsake you. **He Will!**

Whatever we ask according to His will, we shall receive (see Mark 11:23). It is that simple. The enemy is the one who tries to confuse you. He aims to get you confessing something not in God's will or only half in God's will, and he wants you to believe that God's promises didn't work or won't work for you. Remember, the devil is the father of all lies. Your role in all of this is to believe God's Word, receive it and stand fast "with the belt of Truth buckled around your waist" as Ephesians 6:14 (NIV) says.

Believe and confess that you are free—thank Him and praise Him because you know He will do what He says He will. Your confidence is in Him, not in me, not in a process, not in yourself or any others.

Repentance and Renunciation. One thing people often miss (or wish to overlook) is the fact that Jesus Christ is our Lord and Savior. Many people want Jesus as their Savior but not their Lord. Obedience to God is based on our love for God. It is because we love Him and He loves us that we want to go the right way, the Lord's way, the best way. His way is a full life, a free life and an enjoyable life. Those who don't make Him Lord don't realize what they are missing. They are still believing the enemy's lies. Even many Christians today are cheated out of what God has for them because the enemy has blinded them with lies. It is so great and so vital to know that Jesus paid the price with His precious blood for all of our sins and wrongful practices. Yes *all*; it doesn't matter which one, what one, how many or how many times.

Jesus said when we confess our sins and turn from them—repentance and renunciation—He is faithful to forgive us of our sins and cleanse us from all unrighteousness (see 1 John 1:9). "Repent, then, and turn to God," Acts 3:19 urges us, "so that your sins may be wiped out, that times of refreshing may come from the Lord" (NIV).

When we repent, we are choosing to turn from the offense or wrongful practice back to God. What a great and divine exchange! But keep in mind what 1 John 8:36 says, "He who does what is sinful is of the devil, because the devil has been sinning from the beginning. The reason the Son of God appeared was to destroy the devil's works" (NIV). Unfortunately, the world is getting into a habit of calling many things that are destructive practices against God's will (sin) by different names. Sin is labeled a disease, a hereditary problem a person can't help, or an incurable malady. The world system has a whole host of labels and catagorizations that define the spiritual root right out of existence.

Remember, the world system is one of the major systems that the devil manipulates to get people off-track and stuck in a rut. If the devil can get you to believe you cannot do anything about your addiction—you won't. You will live wih it, cope with it and try to medicate it instead of eradicate it. As a result, you will be entangled, bound and walking in the flesh the rest of your life, and it will affect not only you but all those around you.

You might think, *Well, what if it is a generational problem? There is scientific proof that these things run in dysfunctional families!* Good news, even if it is a generational trait or sin, Jesus redeemed us from the curse by what He did on the cross (Galations 3:13) and broke its power through His blood and resurrection. The Holy Spirit is waiting to confirm this in you. We simply confess the sins of our family, renounce any practices that are against God, and ask Jesus to break any hold they have in our lives or our children's lives. This closes the door to any foothold that the enemy may have had on you through generational curses and iniquities.

The Bible is clear:

"Do not give the devil a foothold" (Ephesians 4:27, NIV).

"Stop sinning or something worse may happen to you"
(John 5:14, NIV).

The way in which we give the enemy a foothold is by opening a door (going against God's Way), which allows the devil entry in our lives. Or else we do not close a door that was already opened by us or someone else in our family, so he is in the habit of walking right in. From such footholds, he then expands his impact. You remember the old saying "If you give him an inch, he'll take a mile?" I remember our pastor, Duane Vander Klok, teaching on this point. He said sin often starts out small, but it will always take you farther than you want to go, keep you longer than you want to stay, and cost you more than you want to pay. This is one of the enemy's methods, getting his foot just a little in the door of your life, entangling you in just a little cord of sin, then expanding his hold until he has you all tied up. Better to firmly lock the door on him!

> *Just like the big bad wolf in the three little pigs story, the wolf couldn't come in or blow the house down when it was built with brick. If our house is built on Jesus and no doors are open, the enemy cannot come in and has no place. The truth is; devil cannot possess what is not yielded to him and cannot stay where he is not welcome.*

Remember, there is no condemnation from God related to sin. He simply says turn from it, confess it and walk My way. So start now, start today! It is never too late, it is never too horrible, it is never unforgivable. Make Jesus both Savior and *Lord* in your life, because if He is Lord of your life, you will want to turn away from any wrongful ways and enjoy the good things He has for you.

Grace and Forgiveness. God's grace is always sufficient for whatever we face, whatever circumstance we are in, whatever our situation. The apostle Paul said that no matter his state, he had learned to abase and abound—to be content in all circumstances—for God's grace was sufficient (see Philippians 4:12–13 and 2 Corinthians 12:9). We need to stay in a place of grace. Oh, what a wonderful state to be in—no matter what goes on, we are not affected by it. Why? Because we are full of God's grace and love.

Grace is a powerful defense against the enemy. One of his tactics, as we discussed earlier, is to wound our hearts and drop in a root of feeling or being unloved. From that springs forth a root of bitterness. The wound is real, and the actions of the wounder are wrong. God never says it is okay for someone to wound you in such a way. In fact, He declares that such actions are wrong according to His Word. What He desires us to do, though, is to stay in or step up into a place of grace and forgiveness so He can heal and protect us.

If the enemy can get you to be unforgiving and judgemental to someone for an offense, he has a right to accuse and torment you even if the offense was a serious wrong like some form of abuse. Not that you deserve such torment, but the law of unforgiveness says if we will not forgive others, how can we expect God to forgive us? (See Luke 6:37 and Matthew 6:14–15). It would be a double standard if you were allowed to hold unforgiveness toward others but still have God forgive you. God is not a God of double standards, but of absolute justice and truth.

When we forgive an offense, what happens in the spiritual world is that the devil loses any foothold on us that was there because of unforgiveness or bitterness (see Hebrews 12:15) and the offender is turned over to God and put in His hands to be dealt with. As long as we hold onto the wrong, we are bound to it, the spiritual force behind it, and to the person who did it. God wants us free from it. Remember, forgiveness is not a feeling—it is an act. It is an act done in faith and from the heart. We do it not because it is *deserved* by the offender, just like our own forgiveness from God is not deserved (see Matthew 6:12–15). We forgive others because we want to be in God's mercy and grace—a great place to be! A protected place!

5
WALKING IN FREEDOM, RESTORATION AND HEALING
How to Get Free and Become Whole

In this chapter, we will walk through the foundational steps of getting you free from your addiction, and then we will claim restoration and healing for your heart, mind and body. As we go through this process, hold on to the Truth.

EXAMINE YOURSELF

Examining yourself is the first step in getting free. It can be a difficult step, but it is vital. The Word of God urges us, "Examine yourselves to see whether you are in faith; test yourselves. Do you not realize that Christ Jesus is in you—unless, of course, you fail the test?" (2 Corinthians 13:5, NIV).

You will not fail the test, though, when you invite the Lord to walk beside you in the process! We will do that together in the prayer that follows. And as Paul told the Corinthians, remember "We're rooting for the Truth to win out in you" (2 Corinthians 13:8, MESSAGE). As you pray this prayer and examine yourself and your ways, measure them against the Word of God—*only* the Word of God—because it is absolute Truth. It is the only measure that won't mislead you, won't distract you and will bring you into liberty—life abundant and complete freedom.

Heavenly Father, in Jesus name, I ask you to reveal to me any ways, thoughts or things in my life that are not of You or are contrary to Your Word. (Name them as He reveals them to you, smoking, jealousy, unforgiveness, etc...). Lord, also reveal to me any generational curses and iniquities that may be in my family, things such as idolatry, poverty, sickness, anger, gossip, witchcraft, sexual impurity and anything else that is not of You. Thank you for showing me any areas where I am out of sync with You so that I can deal with them.

REPENT AND EXCHANGE

Now that God has revealed to you those things that are not of Him or are contrary to Him, turn from them, renounce them and ask God to forgive and erase them (whether they are yours or your family's). When you ask for forgiveness and turn from your wrongful ways, then they will not be your downfall anymore and the enemy will lose any foothold he had in your life. Romans 6:11 says, "Count yourselves dead to sin but alive to God in Christ Jesus" (NIV).

> *Lord, I repent of all my ways that are contrary to Your ways. I renounce any family practices contrary to Your Word that I am aware of and even those I am not aware of. They are wrong, and I want nothing to do with them anymore, Lord, I forgive all those who hurt or offended me and step into your mercy and grace. Father, in Jesus' name and by the power of His blood and resurrection; break their hold, destroy every bondage, cut off every curse and wash them away. In Jesus' name I shut the door to them. I was wrong in my response to them, and that I turned to an addiction and to other things instead of turning to You. Forgive me. Deliver me. Jesus, wash me clean with Your blood and make in me a clean heart. A heart that will follow hard after You. Thank You, Jesus. I love You.*

You have now crossed over from death unto life, just as John 5:24 indicates: "I tell you the truth, whoever hears my word and believes Him who sent me has eternal life and will not be condemned; he has crossed over from death to life" (NIV).

The next thing God wants to do, now that you have crossed over, is exchange all the hurts and wrongs for good gifts, gifts from Him. God will show you what is behind your addiction or behavior, and He wants to remove all of the roots that the enemy has tried to plant inside of you. So whatever it is, however many there are, give them all to God to put on His altar. He will burn them up with His consuming Fire. Remember the story of the prodigal son? (See Luke 15:11–32.) The prodigal took his inheritance and spent it on satisfying his flesh; he came to ruin and then came to himself and realized he could not continue this way. He also realized that his father's place was a better place than where he was. So he turned and went to his father and humbly repented. And do you remember what his father did? His father brought out the best robe (which represented righteousness and sonship), placed a ring on his finger (representing covenant and authority), and shoes on his feet (signifying freedom and honor) because his son was alive. This is a parable of what the Heavenly Father wants to do for you - replace the ruin of the flesh and the wounds of the world with His love, His righteousness and His authority, that you may be free, alive, full of faith, hope and love. You will be a sign and wonder to others of His great love.

Jesus, I thank You that You bought freedom, forgiveness, restoration, healing and peace on the cross for me. Heavenly Father, in Jesus name, I exchange my bondage (smoking, drugs, sex, alchohol, anger, food, fear, ect...), sin, addictions, offenses from others, wrongs, pain, unlovingness, abandonment, loneliness, rebellion, bitterness, abuse, and all the rest (whatever roots He shows you that are behind your addiction to exchange) for Your freedom, life, liberty, love, mercy, grace, forgiveness and peace. Devil, in the name of Jesus, any root you tried to plant is removed! I rip off any label you tried to call me that I am not, and you must get out—the yoke of bondage is destroyed and I am a clean vessel for the Lord in Jesus' name. Fill me now, Holy Spirit, with the gifts of my Heavenly Father. Saturate me in the Father's Love and Your presence. I receive His free gifts and ask you to increase them every day. I'm free, I'm free—thank You, Jesus—I am free!

BELIEVE AND RECEIVE

Faith brings into action a principle within our hearts, maintained the evangelist Smith Wigglesworth, so that Christ can dethrone every power of satan. Simply put, faith is confidence in God and His Word. By believing and receiving, we have what we say. It is so important a principle that I want to spend a little time reinforcing this with you. Mark 11:24 says, "Therefore I tell you, whatever you ask for in prayer, believe that you have received it, and it will be yours" (NIV). Everyone who asks according to God's Word and believes it, they *will* receive. This is not sometimes, maybe, or dependent on you earning it—you just line up, believe it and receive it. The enemy wants you to fear or think that it didn't work for you, but as we discussed before, our God never changes. His Word is truth, and you are set free! "Is not my word like fire," says the Lord, "and like a hammer that breaks a rock in pieces?" (Jeremiah 23:29, NIV).

I thank you, Heavenly Father, that my faith is in You and in Your Word. That it is truth, and the truth makes me free. For who Jesus sets free is free indeed according to John 8:36. I thank You, Jesus, that I am dead to sin and alive to God. I am His child with full rights and authority, and I receive all the good things that He has given me and has planned for me. Holy Spirit, awaken me to God's truths and reveal to me all that God is. I believe it and receive it in Jesus' name—Amen.

In the next sections, you will see some major tactics of the enemy to contest your new-found freedom. Yes, he will contest it, because as a free child of God, you are dangerous to him and his evil plans. For each enemy tactic, God has an answer. So stand in liberty on the Truth, stay free and keep walking in freedom.

Your strength is in the Lord God Almighty. The devil will try to play games with you and take you prisoner again, but God has the answer for every strategy the devil tries to employ. Let's look at a few of his tricks and get familiar with God's battle plan to defeat him!

ENEMY TACTIC ONE: RETURN PRESSURE

One of the tactics that the devil will try to trip you with, now that you are delivered and free, is to try to seduce and tempt you back into bondage.

Don't go back to Egypt! I am reminded of the example of the Israelites as they came out of Egypt. Remember, they had been in bondage, enslaved and even sometimes killed by the Egyptians, but God freed them. They came out of Egypt free, loaded down with all of the treasures of Egypt and headed for the Promised Land (a far better place). Once they got into the desert, satan started tempting them with memories of their old life—the meat, the houses, the leeks and onions…and what happened? Some of them started to murmur, complain and cry out, "I want to go back! At least I know what Egypt was like—I'm not sure about the Promised Land!"

When you think about it, it's crazy. Here they were once again a free nation, loaded with the spoils of Egypt, being fed manna from heaven everyday, miraculously protected, their shoes and clothes never wearing out. Ahead of them lay the great Promised Land given to them by God, a land flowing with milk and honey according to Scripture. And some of them wanted to go back into slavery instead of continuing in God's promise?

Let their story be a live example of how satan is going to try to play you. This is a picture of what the enemy is going to try to get you focused on, your circumstance, what you are feeling or the way it was instead of God's promises and your destiny in Him. The devil will try to get you crying to go back to Egypt. Beware! Don't fall for his trick! Don't sacrifice the good things of God for a cheap imitation that destroys and never satisfies. Don't go back!

Rather, according to James 4:7, "Submit yourselves, then, to God. Resist the devil, and he will flee from you" (NIV). Stand and resist—the enemy will flee because he has to. God's Spirit in us is greater than our testing and temptations, and when we ask Him, He is the one who opens the door to our deliverance and closes the door to the enemy.

Don't go back to Egypt! Don't go back to Egypt!

GOD'S ANSWER: STAND IN LIBERTY BECAUSE HE PROVIDES A WAY OUT

One thing that we need to get straight is that we are never tempted beyond what we are able to withstand. First Corinthians 10:13 indicates that, "No temptation has seized you except what is common to man. And God is faithful; He will not let you be tempted beyond what you can bear. But when you are tempted, He will also provide a way out so that you can *stand up* under it" (NIV, italics added). I want to give you a personal example of this as it relates to me:

> *After I was delivered from smoking and my heart healed from the driving wounds, the very first night my flesh cried out so loud for a cigarette. The enemy was tempting me with a massive craving, and it was right before bedtime. I cried out to God and said, "Lord, you know where I am at—if you don't pin me to this bed, I am going to get in my truck and drive a half hour to buy a pack of cigarettes and smoke them! (I was serious—I was in a bad place.) The next thing I remember is a burning heat in my chest, then I didn't wake up until the next morning, and yes, the craving was gone. From then on, I was able to stand and resist any future cravings the enemy brought.*

God provided a temporary way out of my temptation. He will meet you where you are at in your weaknesses. But for Him to answer, we must cry out, ask and stand with Him. I believe that just like each of us has a unique fingerprint, each of us also has a unique voice that God created and *likes* to hear.

I liken it to this: You know the voice of your child. In fact, if that child was in a massive crowd and cried out in pain, you as the parent would hear it! If that child started laughing, you would know where they were and the state they were in. God is just like that—remember, we are His children.

He likes to talk and walk with us. He likes it when we talk to Him, cry out to Him, laugh with Him, and love Him. He wants to hear from you and me today and every day. He wants a relationship with you, a personal one! He loves you—He loves you—He loves you! He will always make a way!

ENEMY TACTIC 2: DECEPTION AND LIES

A second tactic we should be familiar with is the enemy's use of deception and lies. We must guard against being deceived by the enemy and instead stand fast on God's Word. The enemy is a liar—as we said earlier, he is in fact the father of all lies. You can expect that one of his tactics is to feed you a bunch of lies and see if he can tempt you back into being hooked again.

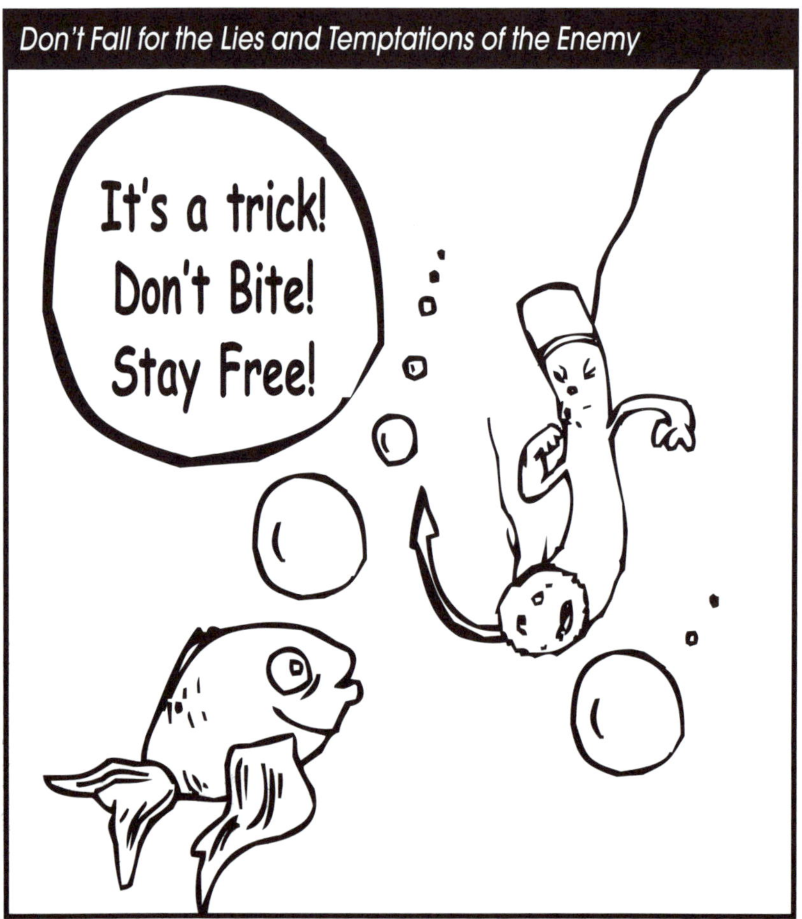

Don't engage your mind in thinking on satan's lies and don't fall for his lies. If you hear any of the following lies, you know they come from the father of lies and his destructive forces:

- ☐ It won't work for you.
- ☐ You are not good enough.
- ☐ God doesn't really care if you have this habit; it doesn't really matter.
- ☐ It is too late.
- ☐ You are not worthy of a call from God.
- ☐ See, the craving is already back—it didn't work.
- ☐ You have never been able to quit before.
- ☐ This didn't really work—it isn't any different.
- ☐ You cannot live without it.
- ☐ No one will know—go ahead.
- ☐ Just one—Just one—Just one—Just one
- ☐ You have done too many things wrong; God doesn't want to use you.
- ☐ You enjoyed it so much—remember the smell, the taste, how you felt
- ☐ Etc…etc…etc…(You get the picture, right?)

GOD'S ANSWER: STAND IN LIBERTY AND PROCLAIM THE TRUTH

So what does God say to do about this pack of lies the devil tries to hook you with? Look at Galatians 5:1: "Stand fast therefore in *liberty* wherewith Christ has made us free, and be not entangled again with the yoke of bondage" (KJV).

Notice where you stand—in liberty, set free. Don't move from where you now stand; you are an overcomer through the blood of the Lamb [JESUS]. How do you make this stand? The Bible says that "You, dear children, are from God and have overcome them, because the one who is in you is greater than the one who is in the world" 1 John 4:4 (NIV).

God is greater than anything the enemy can throw at you, and God lives in you. All of His promises are yes in Christ and through Him amen (see 2 Corinthians 1:20).

Do you know what *amen* means? Amen means "So be it—it is done!" In the book of Revelation, we see that the children of God "overcame him [the devil] by the blood of the Lamb (Jesus) and the word of their testimony" (NIV). So be it! It is done! You stay an overcomer by staying under the blood of the Lamb (Jesus) and proclaiming a testimony of truth, which is from the Word of God. It is settled, it is done; in other words, case closed - no more arguments!

Why do you need to proclaim it as well as believe it and stand on it? Because God's Truth will always overcome the facts of your situation. The fact is the enemy may try to tempt you with cravings, but the truth is you are free and can resist him. God creates the fruit of your lips! In Isaiah 57:19 (KJV), God says exactly that: "I create the fruit of the lips," so what you say going forward is vitally important. (And it's also important to say you are **not** going back!) Proclaim the fruit you believe you will enjoy, even if in the moment things seem difficult. God **will** create your words of truth!

Jesus is always the best example to follow, so let's look at what He did when He was tempted in the desert for 40 days by the devil (see Matthew 4:4, 7, 10 for Jesus' answers to the devil's temptations). The devil tempted Jesus with every temptation known to man, and the Bible clearly shows us how Jesus responded. When the enemy directly tempted Jesus, Jesus' response was, "It is written . . ." *Jesus simply responded to each temptation by declaring the truth that was written in God's Word.* He simply returned God's Word and stood fast, not falling for the enemy's lies and temptations. *God's Word never fails.* Men do, but God's Word never does.

We are to do as Jesus did. You need to stand fast and not fall for the enemy tactics, yet when the enemy comes a-tempting, respond with what is written by God in the Bible. Why? Because God says His Word does not return void and will always accomplish what He sent it to do (see Isaiah 55:11). The enemy doesn't have a chance and has to flee as you stand fast, under the blood of Jesus, proclaiming God's words! It is Living Word—the Word of Truth—accomplishing its Purpose!

ENEMY TACTIC 3: ATTEMPTING TO BREAK YOUR WILL

Another tactic of the enemy is that he wants to break down your will so you become passive and don't resist sin anymore. Realize that he will try and try and try to pound you until you give in. The good news, though, is that we can stand fast against his attacks.

One of your enemies is your flesh, remember. After you get delivered, your flesh is going to speak to you and try to rise above your spirit, which is standing fast on God's Word. Your flesh is going to, in fact, scream at you: "I want a cigarette! I want a drink! I want a cookie!" (or whatever your addiction of choice was). And the devil will tell you that you are not set free because of the way your flesh is reacting.

That's one way he wears you down and tries to break your will—he lies to you about what's happening. Your flesh is having a typical fleshly reaction, but the devil will paint it as some huge spiritual failure on your part. Nothing could be farther from the truth! If you realize his tactic is going to come, then when the flesh and the devil join forces, you will be able to withstand the dual assault. Your spirit will take its rightful place of authority over your flesh and over the devil, commanding it line up with God's Truth and get out! Doing the following things will help you.

GOD'S ANSWER: STAND IN LIBERTY AND RESIST

Purpose in your heart ahead of time to stay free. Determine by an act of your free will that you *will* stay free and *will* not fall back into the habit no matter what. Then when the attack comes, you know which way you will go—with God. No impulsive decisions or wavering; your mind is already made up. You are resolved.

The Old Testament's Daniel is an example of this. He purposed in his heart to follow God and worship only Him no matter what. Later, Daniel was tempted to save his life by worshiping the king instead of

God, lest he face death in the lions' den. It had been decreed that all those who worshiped any god but the king would be put to death. But Daniel's mind had long ago been made up, so what did he do? He worshiped God, as he had purposed in his heart a long time ago. He was not knocked off-kilter by a difficult, in fact a horrible, situation when it suddenly arose. Guess what—God provided a way out when Daniel stood strong against the temptation and chose to go with God. An angel shut the lions' mouths, and Daniel was saved (see Daniel 6).

God will give you the ability to be clear-minded and self-controlled too, no matter what the situation (see 1 Peter 4:7), just as Daniel did in his life-and-death dilemma.

Speak back to your flesh. It is speaking to you, so speak back to it! One of the tactics of the devil is get you to be silent. God's Word is living, and when you speak it out, it accomplishes what it was meant to do in your life! Let it live by speaking it out loud.

As an example of this, suppose your child is headed toward the road, and a big truck is coming toward him or her from the other direction. You can think in your head *Stop!* but that isn't going to affect the outcome of the situation and stop your child. The only way to affect the outcome of the situation is to speak out loud to proclaim to the child *"Stop!"* You have to *say the words* for their power to come into play and make a difference.

It's the same with your flesh. When the flesh speaks, speak back. What do you speak? The Word of God. Get in God's Word and speak the verses of truth that apply directly to your situation. In the back is a set of proclamation cards to help you with this. So speak up, speak out and speak back with the powerful Living Word of God.

Praise and Thanksgiving. Praising God puts you in His presence. Read Psalm 100. Verse 4 says, "Enter His gates with thanksgiving, and His courts with praise: give thanks to Him and praise His name. For the Lord is good and His love endures forever; His faithfulness continues through all generations" (NIV).

Praise also stills the enemy and your avengers (see Psalm 8:2). The Lord actually dwells within the praises of His people: "But thou art holy, O thou that inhabitest the praises of Israel" (Psalm 22:3, KJV). Once you understand that the Lord God inhabits your praises, you can understand why in the Old Testament they typically sent out the musicians and singers before the army. In fact, read over 2 Chronicles 20:21–22, which shows how God inhabited the singers' praise, confused the enemy and laid traps. Think about how many times God used musical methods and worship to run off, confuse or destroy the enemy. The enemy cannot operate in an atmosphere of praise. Here are just a few instances: King David played before Saul and the tormenting spirits left; Israel's enemies turned on themselves and were defeated when Gideon's armies blew the horns and crashed the glass; Jericho's walls fell down at the shout and praise of God's people; and the prison doors flew open for Paul and Silas when they praised God. Praise is powerful, and God likes it and dwells in it. It speaks to how *big* He is. You don't have to be a musician or good singer to praise Him—just thank Him and make joyful noises. Remember, He likes your voice.

Praise shows you have confidence in God and in His Word, because you are thanking Him for the outcome, no matter what the current circumstances look like. Rodney Howard Browne gave the following analogy of Paul and Silas, which I have paraphrased:

> *God was in the heavens listening,*
> *He heard the sounds of praise.*
> *He started tapping his foot to the music*
> *and the jailhouse doors flew open.*
> **Praise brings freedom!**

Joy unspeakable and full of God's glory. (See 1 Peter 1:8). The enemy hates joy and Holy Ghost inspired laughter and joy. Why? Because the devil and his forces cannot operate in it. Why not? Psalms 16:11 says that in the Lord's presence is fullness of joy. So if there is fullness of joy, God's presence is there. The enemy cannot operate in the fullness of God's presence.

Secondly, the joy of the Lord is your strength and a merry heart does good like a cure (see Nehemiah 8:10 and Proverbs 17:22). Even the world understands that laughter in the natural is good for you. Think about it, it feels good to laugh. But we want an even deeper joy than our normal laughter, and God gives us Holy Spirit inspired joy. That's the kind of joy that God bubbles up deep inside us when we step out in faith and laugh and ask Him for it.

Ask the Holy Spirit to fill you with His Joy and just start laughing.

I know there is something very important taking place when you begin this part of the process. Holy joy and laughter break many things in the spiritual and physical realms. I know this because I live it, and God wants happy children. I once heard someone say, that the serious business of heaven is Joy.

Picture this, a good guy (big guy) holding the top of the head of a smaller guy (a little guy), while the little guy is flailing his fists wildly in the air. The Good guy is laughing as all this occurs - showing how big he is and that he knows the little guy can't touch him unless he lets go of him. It is the same in the spiritual realm. Your laughter in tough times, makes a glorious statement of your belief in God's Truth and promises. You are not worried, you won't fail and you know you are on the winning side! God is honored by you honoring how Big and True He is!

Lord let thy will (joy) be done on Earth as it is in heaven.

Encouragement. Find someone who can encourage you in your stand and will agree with you and pray for you. Hebrews 3:13 says we should keep encouraging one another so that none of us is hardened by the lure of sin. If you can't find someone to come alongside you, you can encourage yourself in the Lord. King David did this often, asking his soul why it was so downcast and telling himself to take heart since he would yet live to see God's goodness. It is a good practice to get into whether or not you have others encouraging you. Why not wake up and encourage yourself in the Lord, everyday?

Spiritual Praying. Praying is important and the Scriptures teach us that the fervent and effectual prayer of a righteous man availeth much (James 5:16). There are two levels of prayer: human and spiritual. Human prayer should consist of proclaiming Gods truth, asking, believing and receiving according to His Word. In other words, praying agreement with the Bible and thanking God He will complete it until it does. The second level is spiritual tongues or in other words, the voice of your spirit. It is a gift from God for all according to Luke 2.

Praying in your spiritual prayer language (speaking in unknown tongues) will drive the enemy from your presence. It is the voice of your Spirit talking directly to God. Many people misunderstand spiritual tongues or believe the lies of the devil about this area. If you like Jesus, you'll like the increased presence of the Holy Spirit that tongues represents in you. Jesus and the Holy Spirit are the same, remember. The devil doesn't want you to receive this gift and use it because he knows how powerful it is in you and how detrimental it is to him and his plans for you. It builds you and endues you with power to be able to withstand attack, witness to other people and communicate in a special language that the enemy cannot understand. For example, like when we send computer messages encrypted so only the receiver can decrypt it and read them, spiritual language is an encrypted language to God that the devil cannot decipher. So sing or pray in tongues as often as you can!

Exercising Your Freedom to Choose. You are a free moral agent. Everyone is a free moral agent. That means we get to make choices versus someone dictating to us what we will do. In fact, your life is a series of decisions.Therefore, at the end of the day, you have to make a choice about whom you are going to believe from this day forward.

You have three choices of whom to believe:
God, yourself (mind/flesh) or the devil.

If I were you, I'd go with God. In fact, I have often had to proclaim (in other words scream out at the top of my lungs) "I'm sticking with you,

God, I'm sticking with you!" So stand and be encouraged, you are on the right path. If you were not, satan wouldn't bother to try to get you off the path again, he'd just let his minions sink you deeper into sin.

ENEMY TACTIC 4: YOUR PAST, GUILT AND CONDEMNATION

It happened to the Israelites when they were tempted by their memories of Egypt, and it happens to us—the enemy brings to mind our past. The devil will keep bringing up your past in a couple of ways. First, he will try to tell you who you are based on your past or what you used to do. It is a lie! You are not who you used to be, because God washed it away the moment you repented, believed and accepted Jesus as Lord and Savior: "What this means is that those who become Christians become new persons. They are not the same anymore, for the old life is gone. A new life has begun!" (2 Corinthians 5:17, NLT). God remembers your past no more, so why should you dwell on it? If God doesn't remember your sin and guilt, you shouldn't. Don't live in your past—live in your calling. From a tactical perspective, the enemy is going to try to trigger something in your mind or flesh to make you want to remember and go back to the past. You need to identify what may be likely triggers of your habit or wound. For example, if you used to drink coffee and smoke, you may want to skip the coffee until you're strengthened enough to resist smoking along with it. If stress triggers it, have your verses out and be ready to speak to stress and command it to go in Jesus' name. Or, if you smoked in your car, purpose in your heart before you get in your car that you will not smoke while driving or riding in a car. Take a lollipop along or a straw to chew on instead.

GOD'S ANSWER: STAND IN LIBERTY
BECAUSE YOUR PAST IS GONE

Second Timothy 2:22 tells us to run from anything that gives us evil thoughts and instead stay close to anything that makes us want to do right.Ask God to show you what you need to run from, and then start running! On your way, pray:

Heavenly Father, I thank You that Jesus bought me freedom from any bondage and that You restore and heal any wound the enemy delivers. I ask You now, Lord, to strengthen my inner man (spirit) with Your love, Your power and Your presence. I purpose in my heart to follow You and Your ways, because they are better than the world's ways, and I choose to stand with You, proclaiming Your truth. Holy Spirit, set up a standard so that when the enemy comes in like a flood, I will not be moved because my feet are upon the Rock, Jesus. Holy Spirit, teach me how to identify the tactics of the enemy and help me to stand strong against them, being clear-minded and self-controlled (1 Peter 4:7). Mind, be quiet in Jesus' name! I thank You, Heavenly Father, that I am Your child, that You perform Your word unswervingly, and that I am an overcomer. Pour out Your love on me, Father, and keep me in all my ways. Fill me with Your joy unspeakable. I praise You, I praise You, I praise You, for You are my Lord and King. I thank You not only for what You do, but for Who You are! I love you! In Jesus' name, Amen.

Healing and Help. Jesus came that we might have life and have it more abundantly, says John 10:10. What good news! This also means that not only does God's anointing destroy the yoke of bondage, but that there is also restoration and healing in it. We discussed earlier how the heart wounds can be healed; now let's spend a little time on physical healing as well. Jesus bought us both. According to Smith Wigglesworth, abundant life means that God the Holy Spirit wants to impart to you love, joy, health and compassion—He is waiting to impart life! Look at Romans 4:17, which says the Lord is the "God who gives life to the dead and calls those things which do not exist as though they did" (NIV). God's Holy Spirit, who resurrected Jesus from the dead, is waiting to resurrect health in your physical body as well. He will quicken it and bring life to it.

Jesus Bought Us Health. Remember, Jesus took 468 stripes for our healing (see Isaiah 53:5 and 1 Peter 2:24). He paid the price—your physical healing is bought and done. You just need to receive it and proclaim it. You need to take God's medicine (His Word) as it relates to your healing, tell your body to line up with His Word and thank Him for it—until the day you see it completed. It may happen instantly (miracle), or over time as a healing process. Either way, it will be brought to completion as you keep on believing and confessing the truth. His Word never fails! Pray this in regard to your physical health:

Heavenly Father, I come to You for my healing in Jesus name, for the Bible says You are the Lord my God who heals me. Lord God, I thank You that You baptize with the Holy Ghost and with fire. Lord, I ask for Your purifying fire now to go through my body, purifying and removing anything not of You. In the name of Jesus, toxins, I say depart now. Lungs, Heart, Liver, (name specifically what needs healing) clear and, I speak life to you in the name of Jesus. Lord, as an act of faith, I breathe in your Holy Spirit and life and breathe out anything not of You. (Physically engage in this as an act of faith: Breathe in and out deeply and slowly ten times right now in Jesus' name. Breathe in life and breathe out death in Jesus' name.) I speak to any destruction that was caused by __________ (name smoking or any other health-destroying habit you have taken part in) and I rebuke the work of the enemy in the name of Jesus. Body and mind, be restored by the power of His word and His precious blood. Every cell, organ and function is healed and well in Jesus' name. I thank You, Jesus, that You bought us perfect health by taking those stripes and shedding Your blood. I believe I am healed, and what is complete in the spiritual realm will quickly and supernaturally manifest to the physical realm. In Jesus' name, Amen.

6

BIG GOD✝ BIG FREE®
Free to Fight for Others and Follow God

God is a God of all comfort, according to 2 Corinthians 1:3–4, which says the God of all comfort "comforts us in all our troubles, so that we can comfort those in any trouble with the comfort we ourselves have received from God" (NIV). God has comforted you and brought you into freedom. As one who has been delivered, whose heart and body are healed, you are now standing in liberty. As an overcomer, you can speak from firsthand experience about who God is and what He has done for you. Nobody can argue with your testimony or take it away from you. You know it—you know it—you know it. You are now living proof of the power of God's Word, and no one can dispute that fact!

That's why the enemy does not want you to be healed and delivered, and why he does not want you to be an overcomer with a powerful testimony—he knows it is a powerful witness of what Jesus did that you now have. Others will see your newfound freedom and be drawn to it. They will want to get free for themselves because of what they see in you. And you can be a freedom fighter for God! If you are willing to let God move through you, He can use you to help bring others out of bondage into freedom. But it's vitally important to understand that it is God and His power that do the moving, not you and your own efforts. Let's take a closer look at how it works.

FIRST THINGS FIRST

Stay focused and don't ever lose track of what is most important. The Bible clearly shows us that in Matthew 22:37-39.

First, love the Lord thy God with all your heart, mind and strength. Second, love thy neighbor as thyself. On these two commands hang everything. Keep God first, spend time with Him, talk to Him, listen to Him and walk with Him. As you do this, you will become so full of His love, that you will become more like Him. He wants each of us to be a *living witness,* who know and live the truth, just like Jesus was a living witness to the truth. No one can deny a changed life and freedom that gives the glory to God.

EMPATHY AND COMPASSION FOR OTHERS

Another thing you gain in Christ besides your liberty is a fresh understanding of what it was like to have been there, bound by habits and addictions, but now set free. This is called empathy. You understand, you have been there. Jesus has the greatest empathy possible with us, because He was tempted by and took upon Himself on the cross every imaginable sin, curse, betrayal, wrongful action and bondage. He wrestled with and conquered it all, even murder. But even more importantly than empathy, Jesus has compassion, a compassion that moved Him to do something about fallen mankind and their state. Look in your Bible at the Gospels sometime and notice how each time He saw hurting people in pain, bondage or shame, Jesus was moved with compassion and took steps to change their situation.

The two key words here are *moved* and *compassion (empathy)*. The enemy has a false replacement for compassion called *sympathy*. But sympathy doesn't do anything about a person's situation except make you feel sorry for them. Compassion and empathy take action—they *move* you to do something about the situation and change it. This is a powerful thought, that as a child of God, you can stand in authority to comfort and impact others through your empathy and compassion; knowing what Jesus bought on the cross.

As you reach out to others, remember that it is not you but the Holy Spirit who lives in you who confirms the Word of God. This is exciting news. There is no stress on you to perform or come up with the answers—you just go and do as He says, and enjoy the ride. It is the Father's will and work to help people, not yours in your own strength, and He wants to move through you when you are moved with compassion.

YOUR COMPETENCE COMES FROM GOD

"He has made us competent as ministers of a new covenant—not of the letter [of the law] but of the Spirit, for the letter kills, but the Spirit gives life" (2 Corinthians 3:6, NIV). It is not you who delivers, heals or binds up the broken-hearted—it is God. Our role is to teach and preach the Good News gospel of Jesus Christ and minister the new covenant. The new covenant is spirit that gives life—if we are full of the Holy Spirit, full of God's presence and God's love, it will pour out of us onto others. God takes care of all the rest. This is why we need God-confidence, not self-confidence. We are the ambassadors, or God's order givers. We give the order according to His Word and He backs it!

Teach, preach and confirm the gospel of Jesus Christ by the power of the Holy Spirit (see Romans 15:19). We are to teach and preach God's promises and truths from a position of authority. Then the Holy Spirit confirms this with signs and wonders. God's Word is life and Spirit.

THE HOLY SPIRIT MUST BE IN ALL YOU DO

God does His work here on earth through His Holy Spirit. We can do nothing unless the Holy Spirit is in it. Part of the problem with many Christians today is they want God but not the Holy Spirit. In other words, they want a form of godliness that denies the power of God. We are to have nothing to do with such lifeless forms of religion. Second Timothy 3:5 warns: "For [although] they hold a form of piety (true religion), they deny and reject and are strangers to the power of it [their conduct belies the genuineness of their profession]. Avoid [all] such people [turn away from them]" (AMPLIFIED).

The Holy Spirit is the power and presence of God in the earth. We need to get out of the way and let Him out of the religious box we try to keep Him in. God's ways are higher than our ways, so we need to get out of the way and let Him work. This was difficult for me, as I was used to making things happen on my own. But what a joy! No stress, just rest—I'm along for the ride with my sweet Jesus by my side.

Whatever you do, catch this: *You don't make it happen.* You are not responsible for the result, you are only responsible to do what God tells you to do. He will take care of the rest. You are not responsible for the result! If He urges and says to your spirit, "Go lay hands on that person over there and claim healing in My name," just do it. Faith is not moved by what you see or feel. Let me say it again, *you are not responsible for the result! God is.* What glorious freedom you have as you just relax, fall in love with God and do what He says. As your compassion moves you to step out in faith and help others, pray:

*Heavenly Father, I thank You that You are the one who confirms
Your Word and that it is already written, and it is finished in*

Jesus. Holy Spirit, I repent of putting You in my religious box, and Jesus, I ask that You remove my old thinking and traditions that made Your cross of no effect, and replace it with Your thoughts and ways, so that I have the mind of Christ. Teach me how to be a child of God and receive His Love. I give You control and thank You, Holy Spirit, that You abide in me every day and at all times and that You teach me all things. Lord, I ask for God-confidence instead of self-confidence. Increase my love of You, love of self and love of others. I thank You that You love me and have good things ahead for me. Prepare me.

Holy Spirit, release Your anointing to flow through my hands and put God's words in my mouth to touch others for you. Rather than sympathy, let me show Your empathy and compassion to others and be moved to action to show them Your love. Lord, I thank You that You are the Light of the World and that when light enters, darkness has to flee. I believe that Your light lives in me, so when I enter a room, darkness and the enemy have to leave. Bless Your Holy Name. Amen.

YOUR DESTINY: FOLLOWING GOD

Now that you are out of bondage and restored, you are also free to follow God and pursue your destiny by fulfilling your God-given calling. God created you, and He called you. No one is excluded from this, although there are some who will choose not to acknowledge it. He has a unique and important purpose for each of us. I have noticed something significant in my experiences with individuals who have been damaged the most by the enemy and hit the hardest by his tactics—when they are touched and turned around by God, these people make some of the greatest evangelists and ministers and living witnesses in the world! The most desperate prisoners make the greatest freedom fighters! I believe that category includes those of us whom the enemy has tried to kill and take captive by means of our desperate and even life-threatening addictions.

I truly believe that the enemy attacks those whom he knows can have the greatest impact against his kingdom of darkness. If the enemy can get you into his kingdom, he can stop you from getting into God's Kingdom. Have you ever noticed how addicted people typically have certain types of personality traits such as forcefulness, stubbornness, boldness and liveliness? When God creates us, He originally puts these traits in us to be used for good purposes and for His glory. The enemy then warps these traits to carry us in wrong directions.

God wants to turn those good traits He designed in us toward Him. In other words, He wants us to be bold for Him, be stubborn about clinging to His Word of truth, live life abundantly in faith and without fear, and forcefully pursue Him as we stand unchangeable against the enemy. I once heard someone compare it to having our foot on the gas pedal of God's car of righteousness on the highway of holiness (godliness) to Him. First Timothy 4:8 says "For bodily exercise profits a little; but godliness is profitable unto **all** things, having promise of the life that now is and of that which is to come" (NKJV). The enemy's plan is to get us to misinterpret things and see them through his warped view, but what we need is godliness, which profits in all areas and sets us on course with God's destiny for us.

Here are some revelations to get straight in our minds. They certainly make me want to get on course with God and get on His highway.

- ☐ Holiness is the opposite of Bondage—it is not some religious thing.
- ☐ Freedom is absolute authority to live abundantly—no dog chain here.
- ☐ God wants a relationship, not religion—there is a big difference.
- ☐ God is a loving Father (see John 14:7)—Jesus is just like Him (of Him, in Him).
- ☐ Heaven is a lively place—a perfect place.
- ☐ Faith is the opposite of Fear and Unbelief.
- ☐ God is a God of Adventure and Risk.
- ☐ Fear of the Lord is reverence for Him and His ways—You like what He likes and dislike what He dislikes – for the same reason.
- ☐ God convicts (Hey, beloved child, what are you doing?)—He never condemns.

- ☐ When light enters, darkness has to leave.
- ☐ God likes to laugh and likes us to laugh—so laugh with Him.

How about you? Do these truths leave you hungry for more of God, regardless of what the world, the flesh, and the devil say or do? Do they make you long to get on course with God and travel His highway to fulfill His destiny for you? Following God is not for the weak of heart or the fence riders. It is for truth believers. Think about His disciples, who were so saturated in His love and so committed to the Gospel (Him) that it didn't matter what the world did or said to them. That's a taste of the freedom I want to have, where nothing that comes my way is able to affect me. Each day when I walk out the door, I travel His highway toward my destiny, because I'm a child of the Lord God Almighty!

LIVING IN HIS PRESENCE—DAILY.
FILLED WITH HIS HOLY GHOST TO THE UTTERMOST!
WHAT FREEDOM! WHAT FREEDOM!

We need to press toward the goal, as it says in Philippians 3:12, not just keep pace. I like the way Smith Wigglesworth put this once: "Don't just keep pace, if you are making no headway, you are a backslider." satan wants to stop or decrease your influence any way he can. Don't let him—you are more than a conqueror in Christ Jesus. God has great plans for you. He is the master planner of the universe and in Jeremiah 29:11 He says to you "For I know the plans that I have for you, plans to prosper you and not to harm you, plans to give you hope and a future."

God has a great purpose for you, so be mighty in spirit and full of His power. We can be confident that as we walk out our destiny, God will faithfully complete it until the end (see Philippians 1:6). Since we are confident of this, we need to run the race to receive our crown, a crown that will last forever (see 1 Corinthians 9:24, James 1:12 and Revelation 2:10–11). Don't give up your eternal crown—it awaits you.

Often people will exchange God's plans for fear or for a feeling, or even worse, for a lesser plan from man. Don't exchange your destiny in Him—nothing will compare to God's purpose. It may be different than you expect, but it sure is a grand adventure.

I want to pray for you, my readers, as you follow God and walk in your destiny, free to fulfill His plans for you:

> *Heavenly Father, in Jesus name, I ask that You release Your anointing and gifts in each one of these people. The gifts that You have given them, Lord, to be used for Your glory. Lord, each of us is a special person, with special purposes for this time and place, because You designed each one of us in our mother's womb and You knew us before the foundations of the world were laid. Heavenly Father, you have special things planned for each one that only he or she can fulfill. No one can take their place, so we ask You to begin to reveal their destiny to them. Holy Spirit, rain down the Father's Love for them and saturate them with His presence. We ask that You stir up their destiny and calling; stir it up in them over the next days, weeks and years, and walk it out with them—hand in hand.*

> *Heavenly Father, I also pray a blessing over each one of these people, Your children. Lord, bless them and keep them; Lord, make Your face to shine upon them and be gracious to them. Protect them, Lord, encamp Your angels round about them and protect them like a wall of fire. Be gracious unto them, shine Your countenance upon them and grant them Godly favor and Your peace. I thank You, Lord, that You love them and will never leave them nor forsake them. I praise You and bless You, Lord, for Who You are and what You have done. In Jesus' mighty name, Amen.*

Now that you are free, stand strong in your liberty. I like how Souza put it because I believe his poem lines up exactly with the psalms and with our Father's will being done on earth as it is in heaven:

DANCE—As though no one is watching you
LOVE—As though you have never been hurt before
SING—As though no one can hear you,
LIVE—As though heaven is on earth!

God wants you living completely free here on earth. He wants to hear you sing, watch you dance with joy and give you a new paradigm of what love is.

LIVING IN FREEDOM AND ABUNDANCE

Freedom is a wonderful thing. That is why our Heavenly Father designed us to be Free. Free moral agents. Free from bondage and pain. Free to live an abundant life. Free to spread the good news of Jesus Christ. Free to be His children again.

HE LOVES US,
HE LOVES YOU,
YES INDEED, HE WILL DO
FOR YOU WHAT HE HAS DONE FOR ME,
SET YOU COMPLETELY FREE.
BIG GOD—BIG FREE!

I am so thankful that God is a perfect communicator—He provides simple ways to obtain extraordinary results. Results that come not because of what we do or say, but because of Him and Who He is. The good results you see in your life from reading this book and applying its principles come directly through the power of God's Living Word. "The entrance of Your words gives light; it gives understanding to the simple (Psalm 119:130, NKJV). So in conclusion I proclaim for you in the mighty name of Jesus and by the power of His blood:

Go on to live a godly life, an abundant life, a free life, a long life, a full life! Be the salt of the earth and the light of the world, and claim your blood-bought rights. God's love can go deeper than any root of the enemy, any wound of the world. As you press on from here, my prayer for you is the same as the apostle Paul's prayer for the Ephesians:

> *I pray that out of His glorious riches the Heavenly Father may strengthen you with power through His Spirit in your inner being, so that Christ may dwell in your hearts through faith. And I pray that you, being rooted and established in love, may have power . . . to grasp how wide and long and high and deep is the love of Christ, and to know this love that surpasses knowledge—that you may be filled to the measure of all the fullness of God.*

Ephesians 3:16–19, NIV

Stay rooted and grounded in His love. Keep moving on with God—your crown awaits! See you in heaven some day!

Michelle

P.S. – Don't forget to find your freedom stone (see the Freedom Stone Liberty Toolkit section) and place it where you can see it everyday.

7
FAQs AND A
LIBERTY TOOL KIT

In this final chapter, you will find the answers to the most frequently asked questions about walking through and applying these freedom principles to your life. In addition, you will find a liberty tool kit full of spiritual helps. First is a page of declarations for you to speak aloud every day that signifies your freedom and puts God's living Word into action every day. If you have never declared Jesus as your Lord, there is a section to walk you through that process and help you become a child of God, with full rights to all the blessings of His Kingdom—including freedom! Likewise, if you are new to the gift of spiritual tongues, there is a section to get you started learning about and experiencing that powerful tool God has given us. Additional resources are also listed that I found especially helpful in my walk into freedom. You may find them helpful as well. Another section encourages you to write down your personal story, or testimony, and consider sharing it with others to encourage them and declare the Works of the Lord. Also, I ask you to take another step in finding a freedom stone to remember what God has done for you. Lastly, I have reproduced the ministry prayers that were scattered throughout the pages of this book so you would have them all in one place, easily available for your use. Be blessed!

FREQUENTLY ASKED QUESTIONS

DOES THIS PROCESS WORK FOR ANYONE?

God is no respecter of persons (see Acts 10:34). What he has done for one, He will do for all. He will set anyone free who wants to be free and follows His way.

DOES GOD'S PROCESS WORK FOR THE UNSAVED?

I believe that God will even set free the unsaved. He is a Big God and no respecter of persons. It is God's Power, not the person, that makes all the difference. I believe during His ministry on earth, Jesus healed and delivered many people who were not saved. He didn't ask them to get saved and then deliver them or heal them. I believe He still does the same, though I hope that after Jesus sets an unsaved person free, he or she will reconsider and choose Him as Savior and Lord. The reality is that some people do not. Some that Jesus healed knew Him as their healer, but they didn't follow Him and have a personal relationship with Him - the best part. If you are unsaved, it is a Big open door to the enemy. I would urge you not to let that be the case with you. Turn to the appendix entitled "Do You Want to Make Jesus Your Lord and Savior?" for additional help in this area.

WHAT IF I DIDN'T EXACTLY FOLLOW ALL THE STEPS IN THIS PROCESS?

This is not a legalistic process. If you repented, turned and asked God to forgive and deliver you, He will do it. Mathew 15:6 tells us that the traditions of men make the cross of Jesus of no effect. It is not the process itself, it is not the church, and it is not me that brings you results and freedom. It is God's power and presence when we line up with His Living Word, the Truth.

WHAT IF I SLIP AND INDULGE AGAIN (WHATEVER IT MAY BE)?

I say: Quit until you Quit! Sometimes it is like learning something new, for example riding a bike. Sometimes you fall off. What do you do? Get back on. If you fall out of your newfound freedom, repent, get free again and move on. There is no condemnation in Christ Jesus, remember.

WHAT IF I DIDN'T FEEL ANYTHING AS I WENT THROUGH THIS PROCESS?

Some people feel things and others do not. I believe that you *know* that you are free, though. This type of thought, that it didn't work because I didn't feel anything, is the enemy trying to get you to think it didn't work. Tell the thought to get out in Jesus' name—*you are free!*

DON'T I NEED TO GO THROUGH THIS MORE THAN ONCE? MAYBE MAKE IT A LONGER PROCESS OR MORE TIMES?

No. When God healed or delivered someone in the Bible, He did it once. He is the same today. God may continue to show you more things that He wants you to get free of and exchange. That kind of spiritual growth is a life process. But otherwise, no. One time can settle your freedom from an addiction. The enemy lies to you, trying to get you to think you are still bound, it is still there, it didn't go, you need more times, you need to earn it, and on and on. The devil is a liar! ONCE AND FOR ALL is enough with our Big God!

The second trick the enemy plays here is that he tries to seduce you into being dependent on something or someone other than God. Don't fall for it. Such things will never work; people will pass away and will inevitably let you down. Base your dependence on an eternal, unchanging God, not a human man.

CAN I REALLY PRAY FOR OTHERS AND SEE THEM SET FREE?

Yes, no credentials required. Only Jesus, as your Lord and Savior, and the Holy Spirit living in you. So get out of His way, but make yourself available and start praying with and for others today! He knows who is ready to receive—ask Him to show you who and how.

WHY DO SO MANY CHRISTIANS LIVE IN BONDAGE? EITHER THEY DON'T GET FREE OR THEIR CHURCHES DON'T HELP THEM GET FREE?

The enemy blinds many and tries to keep people ignorant of God's Truth. He doesn't want you to hear it, he doesn't want you to believe it if you have heard it, and he doesn't want you to apply it to yourself or others. This is simply the case. If we know the truth, we should live it, proclaim and practice it and give it to others. The enemy's biggest strategy today is lulling the church to sleep and getting us to deny the power and presence of God and His Holy Spirit. Picture a knight in shining armor with a massive sword, bundled up in a straight-jacket. This is what we are talking about—being of no effect. We are free moral agents and can believe what we want to believe. If one chooses to believe the enemy's lies, it will be difficult to choose to walk into freedom in God's power.

I HEARD THAT SPEAKING IN TONGUES IS OF THE DEVIL. HOW DO YOU REPLY TO THAT?

It is not. If you don't believe me—take it up with God—it's in His Word. He is the one Who gives us tongues and in the Bible, told us to use the gift. You don't have to speak in tongues, but I don't know why you wouldn't want one of God's gifts. They are always good. His disciples always used it. I liken it to the way we encrypt data messages that are sensitive and only to be viewed by certain people. It also resembles the wartime strategy of creating secret codes that the enemy doesn't understand. Our spiritual language is between our spirit and God. The enemy does not understand it, so of course he doesn't want you to have a prayer language or use it. It is powerful. Think on this: When Jesus received the Baptism of the Holy Spirit, the devil panicked and went wild. He knew when the Holy Spirit fills someone, it is a massive blow to his dark kingdom. Spiritual tongues is a sign of a deeper infilling of the Holy Spirit, an enduement of power, in your life.

Now, if you ask someone other than Almighty God and Jesus to give you this language, that is of the devil. Only receive from God, by asking Him in Jesus' name, directly.

WHY DO I NEED THE BAPTISM IN THE HOLY SPIRIT? I THOUGHT I GOT IT ALL WHEN I GOT SAVED!

You did receive the Holy Spirit when you got saved. The baptism, however, is about the continual increase and filling of the Holy Spirit. Just as the disciples needed it, so do you. It is for your edification (building up of your spiritual man) and witness. If you want to witness to others, the Holy Spirit is the one Who confirms the Word of God with signs and wonders, so the more of Him you have, the better. Read Psalm 143:10; John 16; Acts 1, 2, 8, and 19; and the book of Jude.

MY MIND IS FLOODED WITH ALL KINDS OF PESTERING THOUGHTS—WHAT DO I DO?

First, command your thoughts (mind) to be quiet in Jesus' name. Remember, your mind did not get made anew but needs to be renewed with the Word of God (Truth). The enemy can only entice you into his game through your body and your mind, so he attacks heavily in both places. If your thoughts have been his playground, kick him out because he doesn't play fair.

Second, command every thought captive to the obedience of Jesus Christ and cast down every vain imagination (see 2 Corinthians 10:5).

Do this as often as it is necessary. Your spirit is in control of and has authority over your mind.

DOES THIS APPROACH WORK FOR ALL TYPES OF ADDICTIONS (SUBSTANCE ABUSE, ALCOHOL, SHOPPING, FOOD, ETC.)?

Yes, because biblical principles (God's truths) are the same regardless of what you are applying them to, and God wants us completely free in every area. Perhaps some of the details of your situation will be different, and when you take your stand for liberty, you will put into practice different ways of keeping your flesh subdued. If you were a smoker, you may need to stay away from situations in which you smoked. If you were into Internet pornography, you may have to sever your Internet connection or find an accountability partner. If you were a shopaholic, you may have to surrender your credit cards for the time being. There are many and various ways the practical details of this process might play out, but other than that, there is no difference in its application. As I said at the beginning of this book, I have seen this biblically-principled approach work for every type of addiction and bondage. God's Truths are true for every area of our lives.

I CAN BELIEVE THAT GOD WILL SAVE ME, BUT I DON'T KNOW ABOUT HIM HEALING ME—I REALLY DESERVE THE DAMAGE TO MY BODY, BECAUSE I CHOSE TO PARTAKE.

God can and *does* want to heal you. When you repented and asked God to forgive you, He washed away your sin and connected you to a new bloodline, Jesus. God wants heaven on earth for you. He wants His will done on earth as it is in heaven, which means no sin and no sickness either. He wants to both take away your sin and heal you—every cell, every organ and every function you have. Remember, your Kingdom linage as a child of God gave you a full rights package. Full means everything, which therefore means physical healing too. Another way God showed me how to look at this is that healing is freedom from the bondage of sickness—just another part of Jesus setting you free!

DECLARATIONS OF FREEDOM TO SPEAK OUT LOUD EVERY DAY

I've included the following declarations for you as proclamation cards in the appendices. Say these Truths **out loud**, **every day**, multiple times a day (it takes less than two minutes). Say them as often as you can! A set of tear-out proclamations cards are located in the appendix. Post them where you can see them, wherever you used to partake in your addictions or where you need reminders to hold fast to God's Truth instead of triggering into old ways! This is part of declaring who you are in Jesus and how you are now standing free.

Note: Make as many copies as you need

Download an audio version of the declaration to speak along with from the website: www.BigGodBigFree.com

FREE INDEED

If Jesus sets you free, you are free indeed!
(*John 8:36*)

I AM A CHILD OF GOD:
I have turned from my old ways and now Jesus Christ is my Lord and Savior. Therefore, I am a child of the Most High God, with the full rights of a son/daughter.

(Galatians 4:4–5; John 3:16–17)

GOD LOVES ME:
There is no condemnation for those in Christ Jesus. His Spirit of life has set me free. How great is the love God lavishes on me, His child.

(1 John 3:1; Romans 8:1 2)

MY BODY IS GOD'S TEMPLE:
God's Spirit lives in me. My hope is in Him. Therefore, I continually examine and purify myself as He is pure.

(1 Corinthians 3:16; I John 3:3; 2 Corinthians 13:5)

I AM DEAD TO SIN—ALIVE TO GOD:
Jesus, I exchange my addiction for Your Spirit of Love, Liberty, Life and Holiness in Jesus' name. Thank You that my spirit is master over my flesh and that Your Holy Spirit has strengthened my inner man with a will and might to overcome.

(Matthew 18:18; Romans 6:11; I John 4:4)

I AM RESISTING SIN—STANDING ON GOD'S PROMISES:
I submit to God and resist the devil and his works of sin—he flees; for greater is He that is in me than he that is in the world. I will believe God; not myself nor the devil, for God's promises are yes and amen. I'm standing fast in liberty, healed of the Lord, and I will not be entangled again. Jesus paid the price—I receive the promise.

(James 4:7; 2 Corinthians 1:20; Galatians 5:1; 1 Peter 2:24)

I AM RUNNING TO MY GOD-GIVEN DESTINY:
I only want to follow God's plan for my life—for it is good and full of hope. I will run my race, Mighty in Spirit, Full of His Power, Saturated in His love. My crown awaits.

(Jeremiah 29:11; Philippians 1:6; I Corinthians 9:24; Revelation 2: 10 11)

I'M STICKING WITH YOU, GOD!
I WILL NOT TURN BACK!
I WILL NOT GO BACK TO EGYPT!

RECEIVING JESUS CHRIST AS YOUR LORD AND SAVIOR

If you have never given your life to Jesus Christ and asked Him to be your Lord and Savior, I hope that today, you reconsider your position. Why? It is a position that determines your eternal future and where you will spend it. Once you die, it is too late. If you have decided you want to receive Jesus as your Lord and Savior, just pray out loud the following prayer from your heart:

Lord Jesus, I ask you to come into my life today. I'm tired of living my life for myself and I want to live it for You. I turn from my wrongful ways and repent of my sins and iniquities. Forgive me, wash me clean in Your precious blood and come into my heart. I believe that you are the Son of God, who came in the flesh. I believe You were crucified, died and were buried, and that You rose again from the dead. You ascended into heaven and now sit at God's right hand. I believe that You shed your precious blood for the remission of my sins. Heavenly Father, I thank You that You sent Your Son, Jesus, who died for me that I might be forgiven, reconciled to You and become Your child. Jesus, You are now my Lord and Savior, and I thank You that the Holy Spirit will abide in me and walk with me the rest of my life. He will comfort me, help me, teach me and guide me in Your ways. Devil, you just lost me; Jesus, You got me! Thank You, Jesus, in Your mighty name, Amen!

____

(Sign and date this on the line above)

ALL OF HEAVEN IS CELEBRATING!!!

If you just prayed this prayer, contact one of the ministry resources listed later in this book. These ministries would like to share with you some free resources that will help you in your new life with Jesus. If you haven't been water baptized, go and be baptized, as Acts 2:38 instructs: "Repent and be baptized, every one of you, in the name of Jesus Christ for the forgiveness of your sins. And you will receive the gift of the Holy Spirit" (NIV). Be blessed, and I'll see you in heaven some day!

SALVATION THROUGH JESUS CHIRST SCRIPTURES:

And everyone who calls on the name of the Lord will be saved.

Acts 2:21, NIV

That if you confess with your mouth, "Jesus is Lord," and believe in your heart that God raised Him from the dead, you will be saved. For it is with your heart that you believe and are justified, and it is with your mouth that you confess and are saved. As the Scripture says, "Anyone who trusts in Him will never be put to shame." For there is no difference between Jew and Gentile—the same Lord is Lord of all and richly blesses all who call on him, for, "Everyone who calls on the name of the Lord will be saved."

Romans 10:9-13, NIV

For God so loved the world that he gave His one and only Son, that whoever believes in Him shall not perish but have eternal life.

John 3:16, NIV

All that the Father gives me will come to me, and whoever comes to me I will never drive away.

John 6:37 NIV

IMMERSION IN THE HOLY SPIRIT

One of the greatest gifts the Heavenly Father gives us is the Baptism in the Holy Spirit, with the evidence of speaking in unknown tongues. This is a spiritual language—you don't understand it with your human mind, but it is your spirit directly praying and praising through the Holy Spirit to the Heavenly Father. It is the voice of your spirit instead of your mind. This is a gift that helps empower you to live the victorious life of an overcomer. The Holy Spirit is exactly like Jesus, so you want more of Him—everyday. To be baptized in the Holy Spirit, pray this prayer:

Heavenly Father, I thank You that I am Your child and that Jesus is my Lord and Savior. I thank You that You give only good gifts to Your children. You said in Your Word that you give the Holy Spirit to those who ask. Lord Jesus, I come to You in faith and ask You to fill and overflow me now with Your Holy Spirit, the same enduement power that happened on the day of Pentecost. As I take the initiative to speak, I expect that the Holy Spirit will give me unknown syllables or sounds that I will speak out. They may sound unusual or different, they may only be one or two syllables to start, but I know they are from You, Holy Spirit, and I will do my part by opening my mouth and speaking them. I thank You, Lord, for Your Holy Spirit and for the gift of spiritual tongues.

Now, speak or sing the sounds or syllables that He has given you, not in your own language, but how they sound in your spirit language, your beautiful heavenly language. Keep doing this every day, and God will continue to give you more and more. Be filled with the fullness of God (Eph. 3:19) and bodly <u>proclaim</u> the Gospel of Jesus Christ and <u>do</u> the will of our Heavenly Father.

For an increase in spiritual prayer audio clip, go to www.BigGodBigFree.com, and under freedom choices.

BAPTISM IN THE HOLY SPIRIT AND SPEAKING IN TONGUES SCRIPTURES:

If you then, though you are evil, know how to give good gifts to your children, how much more will your Father in heaven give the Holy Spirit to those who ask him!

Luke 11:13, NIV

All of them were filled with the Holy Spirit and began to speak in other tongues as the Spirit enabled them.

Acts 2:4, NIV

And I will ask the Father, and he will give you another Counselor to be with you forever—the Spirit of truth. The world cannot accept him, because it neither sees him nor knows him. But you know him, for he lives with you and will be in you.

John 14:16-17, NIV

However, as it is written: "No eye has seen, no ear has heard, no mind has conceived what God has prepared for those who love him"—but God has revealed it to us by his Spirit.

The Spirit searches all things, even the deep things of God. For who among men knows the thoughts of a man except the man's spirit within him? In the same way no one knows the thoughts of God except the Spirit of God. We have not received the spirit of the world but the Spirit who is from God, that we may understand what God has freely given us. This is what we speak, not in words taught us by human wisdom but in words taught by the Spirit, expressing spiritual truths in spiritual words.

1 Corinthians 2:9–13, NIV

In the same way, the Spirit helps us in our weakness. We do not know what we ought to pray for, but the Spirit himself intercedes for us with groans that words cannot express.

Romans 8:26, NIV

But you, dear friends, build yourselves up in your most holy faith and pray in the Holy Spirit.

Jude 20, NIV

And these signs shall follow those who believe; in my name they shall cast out demons, they shall speak with new tounges.

Mark 16-17, NKJV

Praying always with all prayer and supplication in the Spirit…

Ephesians 6:18, KJV

See also:

Luke 24:49; Eph. 3:19; Eph. 5:18-19; Acts 1:4-8; 1st Corinthians 14; and Isaiah 28:11-12

Ministries / Prayer Lines

The following ministries have prayer lines that you may call when you want someone to pray with you. These ministries adhere to biblical principles and will pray in faith with you, adhering to the truth and the Word of God.

Kenneth Copeland Ministries*   800-600-7395

Kenneth Hagin – Word of Faith Ministries*   918-258-1588

Resurrection Life Church—Walking by Faith*   616-261-9000

Prayer of Agreement Audio Clip: www.BigGodBigFree.com
Under Freedom Choices

**The listing of these ministries does not mean they support or endorse this book or by desiGn ministries, inc in any way. They are some of the author's personal favorites.*

ADDITIONAL RESOURCES

Listed here are a few resources that I have found very helpful in the journey of life and walking out my new freedom. Others have found them helpful, too, so perhaps you will as well. I have organized them by type of resource to assist you.

Music / Books / CDs

Father Heart Communications*—I recommend their CD and resources related to *The Father's Love Letter.* It is a message to saturate yourself in as you begin to understand the love that the Heavenly Father has for you. Website:
http://www.Fathersloveletter.com

James and Teresa Jordan*—Out of New Zealand and Father Heart Ministries, these two have wonderful resources on the Heavenly Father and His love. Their topics range from the Father's Spirit of Adoption and Sonship to the Father's Freedom, and so forth. Their resources are listed on their website: *http://www.fatherheart.net*

Jesse Duplantis Ministries*—Out of New Orleans, this ministry has wonderful resources that will lift your heart and help you grow your spirit. My favorite is God isn't a God of Enough - He's too Much and Close Encounters of the God Kind. Check out their resources on their website: *http://www.jdm.org*

by desiGn ministries, inc.—The website includes ministry prayers, teachings and ecouragment audio clips (listen on–line or download) as well as other liberty resources and helpful hints related to getting free and standing in freedom. *http://www.BigGodBigFree.com* or *http://www.bydesignministries.org*

Jerry Savelle Ministries*—Home of the Chariots of Light Bikers Club at *http://www.jerrysavelle.org*

*The listing of these ministries does not mean they support or endorse this book or by desiGn ministries, inc in any way.
They are some of the author's personal favorites.*

YOUR PERSONAL TESTIMONY

I have provided an area for you to write and to declare your personal testimony about how the Lord has set you free. Take time to fill it out, and then keep it as a memorial to this great day in your life. If you have moments of doubt or temptation, pull it out and read it to remind yourself that you are a child of God and heir to all the riches, blessings, and benefits of freedom and abundant life we have talked about within these pages! Or share it with a friend or relative who is seeking to walk out of bondage and into freedom. Give them a copy so they can remind themselves of what God has done for you, and make sure they know that He is no respecter of persons—what He has done for you, He will freely do for them, too!

SHARE YOUR TESTIMONY TO ENCOURAGE OTHERS

If you would like to allow me to share your testimony as a way of encouraging others and giving them hope, please check the box below and send me a copy of your testimony page and this page at the address below.

___ Yes, you may use part or all of my testimony (only first names will be used unless otherwise requested) to declare the works of the Lord! I understand it may be publicly displayed.

Check the above box and send your testimony to the address shown below, or go online at www.bydesignministries.org and write your testimony there.

by desiGn ministries, inc.
P.O. Box 122
Clarksville, MI 48815

MY TESTIMONY

I will proclaim what God has done for me. I will "declare His glory among the nations, His marvelous deeds among all peoples" (Psalm 96:3, NIV). For I overcome the enemy by the Blood of the Lamb (Jesus) and the words of my testimony (Rev 12:11):

____

____

____

____

____

____

____

____

____

____

____

____

____

____

____

I am a living witness to what Jesus Christ has done:

____
(fill in your name and the date)

FREEDOM STONE

I want you to participate in one more step that declares and signifies your new found freedom in Jesus Christ. Read Joshua Chapter 4 which describes when the Israelites finally crossed the river into the Promised Land God had given them. In particular, read verses 4-10 and 21-24. God had them gather and place stones so that future generations and others would inquire what the stones were for. The Israelites were to declare the mighty hand of God and what He had done for them, when people or their children inquired of these stones and their purpose. So read the chapter and then complete the following.

Find a stone, it can be any size, shape, color, etc. and find a place to put it. The place you put this stone should be somewhere where you will see it everyday and where others will see it. Why? So that you are reminded of how God freed you and when others inquire, you are able to tell them of the wonderful freedom working God you have.

When you see the stone – Thank God for the great things He has done for you! Joshua 4:24 says:

> *That all the people of the earth might know the hand of the Lord, that it is mighty; that ye might fear the Lord your God forever.*

MINISTRY SECTIONS FROM THE BOOK

What follows are the prayers that were spaced throughout the book. Here they are all printed in one location for easy reference. Pray them from your heart and pray them over others as you minister

INVITATION AND OPENING PRAYER

I would like to open your reading with the following prayer (please pray this out loud):

> **Pg. xii -** *Heavenly Father, in the name of Jesus, we welcome You to this place and into our lives. Holy Spirit, we ask that*

You prepare and open our hearts to receive the powerful and living Word of the Lord. Remove any thinking that isn't in agreement with God's ways and open our spiritual eyes and ears to hear and receive. We welcome You to heal, restore and deliver us; to touch our hearts, our minds, our emotions and our bodies today, in the name of Jesus. We thank You, Lord Jesus, for Your death and resurrection. It is Your blood that cleanses us from our unrighteousness and restores us. We speak to fear, anxiety and any enemy forces and render you useless in the name of Jesus. Father, release Your Holy Spirit of Life, Love, Liberty and Adoption to flow freely in our lives from this day forward. Lord, touch us with Your presence, in the name of Jesus Christ, Amen.

Pg. 40 - *Heavenly Father, in Jesus name, I ask You to reveal to me any ways, thoughts or things in my life that are not of You or are contrary to Your Word. (Name them as He reveals them to you, like smoking, jealousy, unforgiveness, etc...). Lord, also reveal to me any generational curses and iniquities that may be in my family, things such as idolatry, poverty, sickness, anger, gossip, witchcraft, sexual impurity and anything else that is not of You. Thank You for showing me any areas where I am out of sync with You so that I can deal with them.*

Pg. 41 - *Lord, I repent of all my ways that are contrary to Your ways. I renounce any family practices contrary to Your Word that I am aware of and even those I am not aware of. They are wrong, and I want nothing to do with them anymore. Lord I forgive all those who hurt or offended me and step into your mercy and grace. Father, in Jesus' name and by the power of His blood and resurrection; break their hold, destroy every bondage, cut-off every curse and wash them away. In Jesus' name I shut the door to them. I was wrong in my response to them, and that I turned to an addiction and to other things instead of turning to You. Forgive me. Deliver me. Jesus, wash* *me clean with Your blood and make in me a clean heart. A heart that will follow hard after You. Thank You, Jesus. I love You.*

Pg. 42 - *Jesus, I thank You that You bought freedom, forgiveness, restoration, healing and peace on the cross for me. Heavenly Father, in Jesus name, I exchange my bondage (smoking, drugs, sex, alchohol, anger, fear, food, ect...), sin, addictions, offenses from others, wrongs, pain, unlovingness, abandonment, loneliness, rebellion, bitterness, abuse and all the rest (whatever He shows you to exchange) for Your freedom, life, liberty, love, mercy, grace, forgiveness and peace. Devil, in the name of Jesus, any root you tried to plant is removed! I rip off any label you tried to call me that I am not, and you must get out—the yoke of bondage is destroyed and I am a clean vessel for the Lord. Fill me now, Holy Spirit, with the gifts of my Heavenly Father. Saturate me in the Father's Love and Your presence. I receive His free gifts and ask you to increase them every day. I'm free, I'm free—thank You, Jesus—I am free!*

Pg. 43 - *I thank you, Heavenly Father, that my faith is in You and in Your Word. That it is truth, and the truth makes me free. For who Jesus sets free is free indeed according to John 8:36. I thank You, Jesus, that I am dead to sin and alive to God. I am His child with full rights and authority, and I receive all the good things that He has given me and has planned for me. Holy Spirit, awaken me to God's truths and reveal to me all that God is. I believe it and receive it in Jesus' name—Amen.*

Pg. 52 - *Ask the Holy Spirit to fill you with His Joy and just start laughing.*

Pg. 55 - *Heavenly Father, I thank You that Jesus bought me freedom from any bondage and that You restore and heal any wound the enemy delivers. I ask You now, Lord, to* strengthen my inner man (spirit) with Your love, Your power and Your presence. I purpose in my heart to follow You and Your ways, because they are better than the world's ways, and I choose to stand with You, proclaiming Your truth. Holy Spirit, set up a standard so that when the enemy comes in like a flood, I will not be moved because my feet are upon the Rock, Jesus. Holy Spirit, teach me how to identify the tactics of the enemy and help me to stand strong against them, being clear-minded and self-controlled (1 Peter 4:7). Mind, be quiet in Jesus' name! I thank You, Heavenly Father, that I am Your child, that You perform Your word unswervingly, and that I am an overcomer. Pour out Your love on me, Father, and keep me in all my ways. Fill me with Your joy unspeakable. I praise You, I praise You, I praise You, for You are my Lord and King. I thank You not only for what You do, but for Who You are! I love you! In Jesus' name, Amen.

Pg. 56 - Heavenly Father, I come to you for my healing in Jeusus name, for the Bible says You are the Lord my God who heals me. Lord God, I thank You that You baptize with the Holy Ghost and with fire. Lord, I ask for Your purifying fire now to go through my body, purifying and removing anything not of you. In the name of Jesus, toxins, I say depart now. Lungs, heart, liver (name specifically) clear and, I speak life to you in the name of Jesus. Lord, as an act of faith, I breathe in your Holy Spirit and life and breathe out anything not of You. (Physically engage in this as an act of faith: Breathe in and out deeply and slowly ten times right now in Jesus' name. Breathe in life and breathe out death in Jesus' name.) I speak to any destruction that was caused by ___ (name smoking or any other health-destroying habit you have taken part in) and I rebuke the work of the enemy in the name of Jesus. Body and mind, be restored by the power of His word and His precious blood. Every cell, organ and function is healed and well in Jesus' name. I thank You, Jesus, that You *bought us perfect health by taking those stripes and shedding Your blood. I believe I am healed, and what is complete in the spiritual realm will quickly and supernaturally manifest to the physical realm. In Jesus' name, Amen.*

Pg. 60 - *Heavenly Father, I thank You that You are the one who confirms Your Word and that it is already written, and it is finished in Jesus. Holy Spirit, I repent of putting You in my religious box, and Jesus, I ask that You remove my old thinking and any traditions that make your cross of no effect, and replace it with Your thoughts and ways, so that I have the mind of Christ. Teach me how to be a child of God and receive His Love. I give You control and thank You, Holy Spirit, that You abide in me every day and at all times and that You teach me all things. Lord, I ask for God-confidence instead of self-confidence. Increase my love of You, love of self and love of others. I thank You that You love me and have good things ahead for me. Prepare me.*

Holy Spirit, release Your anointing to flow through my hands and put God's words in my mouth to touch others for you. Rather than sympathy, let me show your empathy and compassion to others and be moved to action, to show them Your love. Lord, I thank You that You are the Light of the World and that when light enters, darkness has to flee. I believe that Your light lives in me, so when I enter a room, darkness and the enemy have to leave. Bless Your Holy Name. Amen.

Pg. 64 - *Heavenly Father, in Jesus name, I ask that You release Your annointing and gifts in each one of these people. The gifts that You have given them, Lord, to be used for Your glory. Lord, each of us is a special person, with special purposes for this time and place, because You designed each one of us in our mother's womb and You knew us before the foundations of* *the world were laid. Heavenly Father, you have special things planned for each one that only he or she can fulfill. No one can take their place, so we ask You to begin to reveal their destiny to them. Holy Spirit, rain down the Father's Love for them and saturate them with His presence. We ask that You stir up their destiny and calling; stir it up in them over the next days, weeks and years, and walk it out with them—hand in hand. Heavenly Father, I also pray a blessing over each one of these people, Your children. Lord, bless them and keep them; Lord, make Your face to shine upon them and be gracious to them. Protect them, Lord, encamp Your angels round about them and protect them like a wall of fire. Be gracious unto them, shine Your countenance upon them and grant them Godly favor and Your peace. I thank You, Lord, that You love them and will never leave them nor forsake them. I praise You and bless You, Lord, for Who You are and what You have done. In Jesus' mighty name, Amen.*

Pg. 66 - *I pray that out of His glorious riches the Heavenly Father may strengthen you with power through His Spirit in your inner being, so that Christ may dwell in your hearts through faith. And I pray that you, being rooted and established in love, may have power . . . to grasp how wide and long and high and deep is the love of Christ, and to know this love that surpasses knowledge—that you may be filled to the measure of all the fullness of God.*

Ephesians 3:16–19, NIV

He loves us, He loves you, Yes indeed, He will do
For you what He has done for me,
Set you completely Free. Big God—Big Free!

**FREEDOM! FREEDOM!
FREEDOM IN JESUS!
FREEDOM! FREEDOM!
BIG GOD—BIG FREE!**

LIST OF APPENDICES

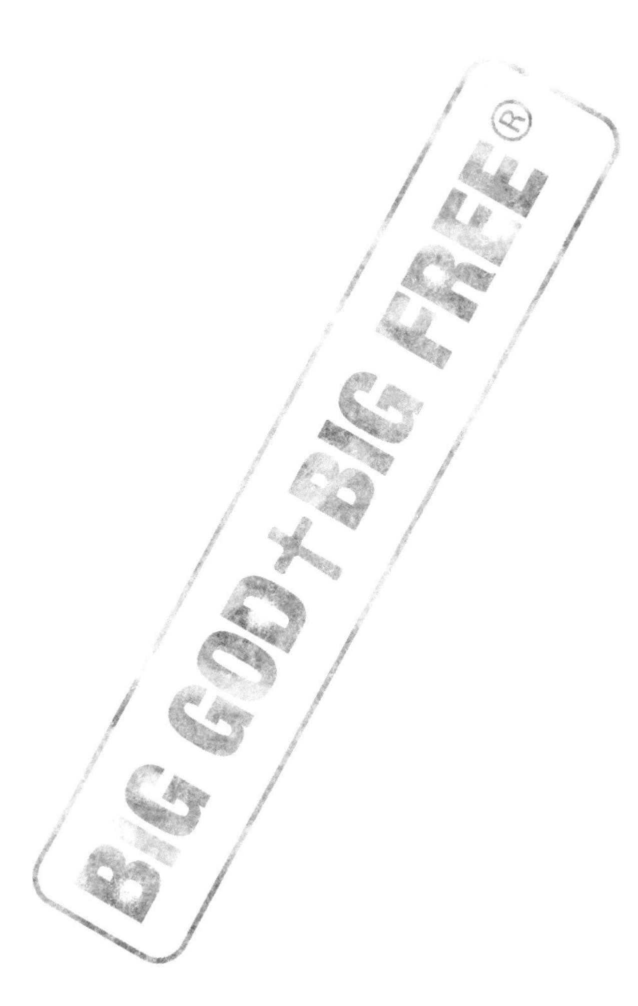

BIG GOD†BIG FREE®

FREE INDEED

If Jesus sets you free, you are free indeed!
(John 8:36)

I AM A CHILD OF GOD:

I have turned from my old ways and now Jesus Christ is my Lord and Savior. Therefore, I am a child of the Most High God, with the full rights of a son/daughter.

(Galatians 4:4–5; John 3:16–17)

GOD LOVES ME:

There is no condemnation for those in Christ Jesus. His Spirit of life has set me free. How great is the love God lavishes on me, His child.

(1 John 3:1; Romans 8:1 2)

MY BODY IS GOD'S TEMPLE:

God's Spirit lives in me. My hope is in Him. Therefore, I continually examine and purify myself as He is pure.

(1 Corinthians 3:16; I John 3:3; 2 Corinthians 13:5)

I AM DEAD TO SIN—ALIVE TO GOD:

Jesus, I exchange my addiction for Your Spirit of Love, Liberty, Life and Holiness in Jesus' name. Thank You that my spirit is master over my flesh and that Your Holy Spirit has strengthened my inner man with a will and might to overcome.

(Matthew 18:18; Romans 6:11; I John 4:4)

I AM RESISTING SIN—STANDING ON GOD'S PROMISES:

I submit to God and resist the devil and his works of sin—he flees; for greater is He that is in me than he that is in the world. I will believe God; not myself nor the devil, for God's promises are yes and amen. I'm standing fast in liberty, healed of the Lord, and I will not be entangled again. Jesus paid the price—I receive the promise.

(James 4:7; 2 Corinthians 1:20; Galatians 5:1; 1 Peter 2:24)

I AM RUNNING TO MY GOD-GIVEN DESTINY:

I only want to follow God's plan for my life—for it is good and full of hope. I will run my race, Mighty in Spirit, Full of His Power, Saturated in His love. My crown awaits.

(Jeremiah 29:11; Philippians 1:6; I Corinthians 9:24; Revelation 2: 10 11)

I'M STICKING WITH YOU, GOD!
I WILL NOT TURN BACK!
I WILL NOT GO BACK TO EGYPT!

www.BigGodBigFree.com

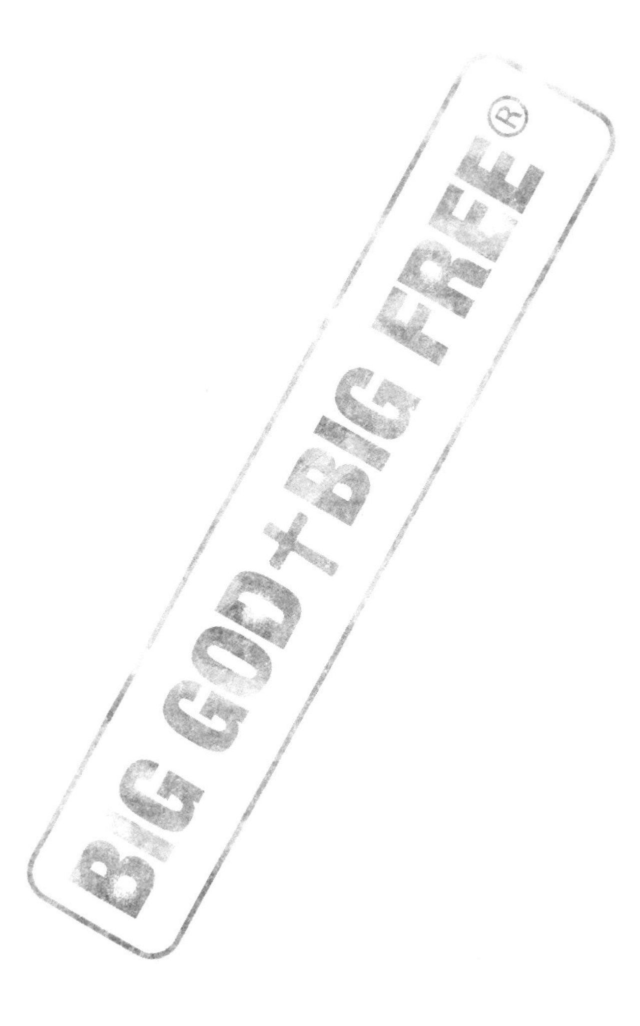

BIG GOD † BIG FREE ®

FREE INDEED

If Jesus sets you free, you are free indeed!
(John 8:36)

I AM A CHILD OF GOD:

I have turned from my old ways and now Jesus Christ is my Lord and Savior. Therefore, I am a child of the Most High God, with the full rights of a son/ daughter.

(Galatians 4:4–5; John 3:16–17)

GOD LOVES ME:

There is no condemnation for those in Christ Jesus. His Spirit of life has set me free. How great is the love God lavishes on me, His child.

(1 John 3:1; Romans 8:1 2)

MY BODY IS GOD'S TEMPLE:

God's Spirit lives in me. My hope is in Him. Therefore, I continually examine and purify myself as He is pure.

(1 Corinthians 3:16; I John 3:3; 2 Corinthians 13:5)

I AM DEAD TO SIN—ALIVE TO GOD:

Jesus, I exchange my addiction for Your Spirit of Love, Liberty, Life and Holiness in Jesus' name. Thank You that my spirit is master over my flesh and that Your Holy Spirit has strengthened my inner man with a will and might to overcome.

(Matthew 18:18; Romans 6:11; I John 4:4)

I AM RESISTING SIN—STANDING ON GOD'S PROMISES:

I submit to God and resist the devil and his works of sin—he flees; for greater is He that is in me than he that is in the world. I will believe God; not myself nor the devil, for God's promises are yes and amen. I'm standing fast in liberty, healed of the Lord, and I will not be entangled again. Jesus paid the price—I receive the promise.

(James 4:7; 2 Corinthians 1:20; Galatians 5:1; 1 Peter 2:24)

I AM RUNNING TO MY GOD-GIVEN DESTINY:

I only want to follow God's plan for my life—for it is good and full of hope. I will run my race, Mighty in Spirit, Full of His Power, Saturated in His love. My crown awaits.

(Jeremiah 29:11; Philippians 1:6; I Corinthians 9:24; Revelation 2: 10 11)

I'M STICKING WITH YOU, GOD!
I WILL NOT TURN BACK!
I WILL NOT GO BACK TO EGYPT!

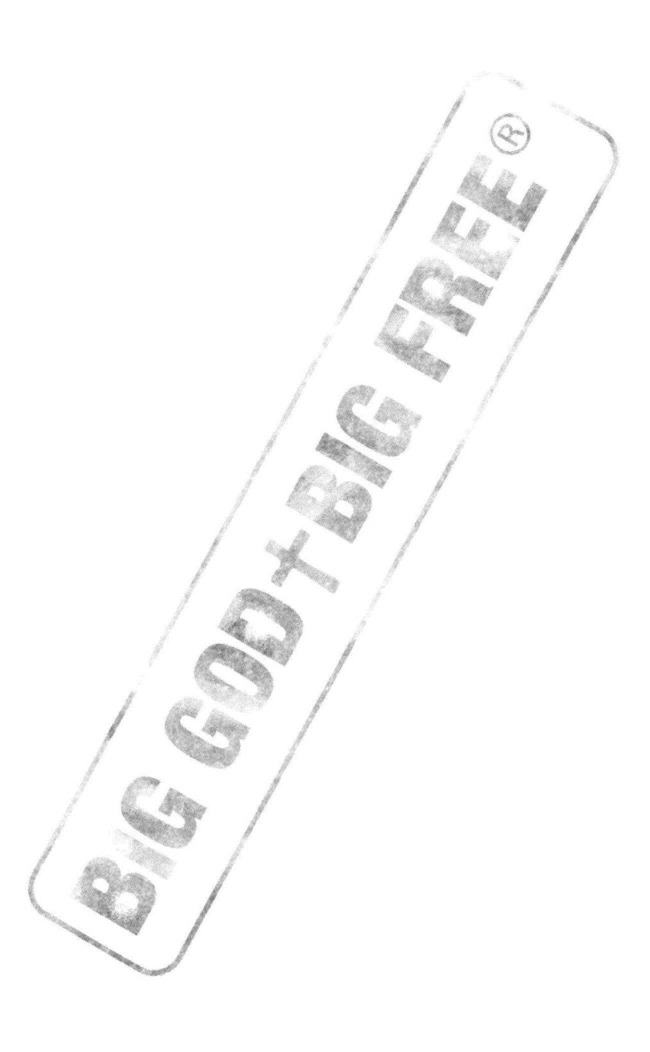

BIG GOD † BIG FREE ®

FREE INDEED

If Jesus sets you free, you are free indeed!
(John 8:36)

I AM A CHILD OF GOD:

I have turned from my old ways and now Jesus Christ is my Lord and Savior. Therefore, I am a child of the Most High God, with the full rights of a son/ daughter.

(Galatians 4:4–5; John 3:16–17)

GOD LOVES ME:

There is no condemnation for those in Christ Jesus. His Spirit of life has set me free. How great is the love God lavishes on me, His child.

(1 John 3:1; Romans 8:12)

MY BODY IS GOD'S TEMPLE:

God's Spirit lives in me. My hope is in Him. Therefore, I continually examine and purify myself as He is pure.

(1 Corinthians 3:16; I John 3:3; 2 Corinthians 13:5)

I AM DEAD TO SIN—ALIVE TO GOD:

Jesus, I exchange my addiction for Your Spirit of Love, Liberty, Life and Holiness in Jesus' name. Thank You that my spirit is master over my flesh and that Your Holy Spirit has strengthened my inner man with a will and might to overcome.

(Matthew 18:18; Romans 6:11; I John 4:4)

I AM RESISTING SIN—STANDING ON GOD'S PROMISES:

I submit to God and resist the devil and his works of sin—he flees; for greater is He that is in me than he that is in the world. I will believe God; not myself nor the devil, for God's promises are yes and amen. I'm standing fast in liberty, healed of the Lord, and I will not be entangled again. Jesus paid the price—I receive the promise.

(James 4:7; 2 Corinthians 1:20; Galatians 5:1; 1 Peter 2:24)

I AM RUNNING TO MY GOD-GIVEN DESTINY:

I only want to follow God's plan for my life—for it is good and full of hope. I will run my race, Mighty in Spirit, Full of His Power, Saturated in His love. My crown awaits.

(Jeremiah 29:11; Philippians 1:6; I Corinthians 9:24; Revelation 2: 10 11)

I'M STICKING WITH YOU, GOD!
I WILL NOT TURN BACK!
I WILL NOT GO BACK TO EGYPT!

BIG GOD†BIG FREE®

BIBLICAL REFERENCES

This is a listing of the biblical references that were used in the book. They are provided for your benefit, in case you do not have a Bible yet. If you don't have a Bible, though, get one! You strengthen your spirit through God's Word. Just as you eat food three times a day to strengthen your body, you need to feed your spirit, too—it eats the Word of God and is built up by spiritual tongues that edify it.

INTRODUCTION

And you shall know the truth, and the truth shall make you free.
John 8:32, NKJV

The Spirit gives life; the flesh counts for nothing. The words I have spoken to you are spirit and they are life.
John 6:63, NIV

No temptation has seized you except what is common to man. And God is faithful; he will not let you be tempted beyond what you can bear. But when you are tempted, he will also provide a way out so that you can stand up under it.
1 Corinthians 10:13, NIV

"For I know the plans I have for you," declares the Lord, "plans to prosper you and not to harm you, plans to give you hope and a future."
Jeremiah 29:11, NIV

CHAPTER 1: WHO AM I?
UNDERSTANDING YOUR MAKER'S DESIGN

O Lord, you have searched me and you know me.
You know when I sit and when I rise;
you perceive my thoughts from afar.
You discern my going out and my lying down;
you are familiar with all my ways.
Before a word is on my tongue
you know it completely, O Lord.
You hem me in—behind and before;
you have laid your hand upon me.
Such knowledge is too wonderful for me,
too lofty for me to attain.
Where can I go from your Spirit?
Where can I flee from your presence?
If I go up to the heavens, you are there;
If I make my bed in the depths, you are there.
If I rise on the wings of the dawn,
if I settle on the far side of the sea,
even there your hand will guide me,
your right hand will hold me fast.
If I say, "Surely the darkness will hide me
and the light become night around me,"
even the darkness will not be dark to you;
the night will shine like the day,
for darkness is as light to you.
For you created my inmost being;
you knit me together in my mother's womb.
I praise you because I am fearfully and wonderfully made;
your works are wonderful, I know that full well.
My frame was not hidden from you
when I was made in the secret place.
When I was woven together in the depths of the earth,
your eyes saw my unformed body.
All the days ordained for me
were written in your book
before one of them came to be.
How precious to me are your thoughts, O God!
How vast is the sum of them!
Were I to count them,
they would outnumber the grains of sand.
When I awake, I am still with you.
Psalm 139:1–18, NIV

But when the time had fully come, God sent his Son, born of a woman, born under law, to redeem those under law, that we might receive the full rights of sons.
Galatians 4:4–5, NIV

For God so loved the world that He gave His only begotten Son, that whoever believes in Him should not perish but have everlasting life. For God did not send His Son into the world to condemn the world, but that the world through Him might be saved.
John 3:16–17, NKJV

Then I heard a loud voice in heaven say: "Now have come the salvation and the power and the kingdom of our God, and the authority of his Christ. For the accuser of our brothers [the devil], who accuses them before our God day and night, has been hurled down."
Revelation 12:10, NIV

Therefore, there is now no condemnation for those who are in Christ Jesus, because through Christ Jesus the law of the Spirit of life ***set me free*** from the law of sin and death.
Romans 8:1–2, NIV (italics added)

And if the Spirit of him who raised Jesus from the dead is living in you, he who raised Christ from the dead will also give life to your mortal bodies through his Spirit, who lives in you.
Romans 8:11, NIV

Do not conform any longer to the pattern of this world, but be transformed by the renewing of your mind. Then you will be able to test and approve what God's will is—his good, pleasing and perfect will.
Romans 12:2, NIV

With my mind I myself serve the law of God, but with the flesh the law of sin.
Romans 7:25, NKJV

Don't you know that you yourselves are God's temple and that God's Spirit lives in you?
1 Corinthians 3:16, NIV

And everyone who has this hope in Him [Jesus] purifies himself, just as He is pure.
1 John 3:3, NKJV

Do you not know that in a race all the runners run, but only one gets the prize? Run in such a way as to get the prize.

Everyone who competes in the games goes into strict training. They do it to get a crown that will not last; but we do it to get a crown that will last forever. Therefore . . . I beat my body and make it my slave so that after I have preached to others, I myself will not be disqualified for the prize.
1 Corinthians 9:24–27 NIV

Let us throw off everything that hinders and the sin that so easily entangles, and let us run with perseverance the race marked out for us. Let us fix our eyes on Jesus, the author and perfecter of our faith . . .
Hebrews 12:1–2, NIV

Blessed is the man who perseveres under trial, because when he has stood the test, he will receive the crown of life that God has promised to those who love him.
James 1:12, NIV

Do not be afraid of what you are about to suffer. I tell you, the devil will put some of you in prison to test you, and you will suffer persecution for ten days. Be faithful, even to the point of death, and I will give you the crown of life. He who has an ear, let him hear what the Spirit says to the churches. He who overcomes will not be hurt at all by the second death.
Revelation 2:10–11, NIV

Even though I walk
through the valley of the shadow of death,
I will fear no evil,
for you are with me;
your rod and your staff,
they comfort me.
Psalm 23:4, NIV

CHAPTER 2: WHOSE AM I?
AMAZING TRUTHS ABOUT YOUR MAKER

If you really knew me, you would know my Father as well. From now on, you do know him and have seen him.
John 14:7, NIV

How great is the love the Father has lavished on us, that we should be called children of God! And that is what we are! . . .
1 John 3:1, NIV

Then said the Lord unto me, Thou hast well seen: for I will hasten my word to perform it.
Jeremiah 1:12, KJV

In the beginning was the Word, and the Word was with God, and the Word was God.
John 1:1, NIV

For the word of God is living and powerful, and sharper than any two-edged sword, piercing even to the division of soul and spirit, and of joints and marrow, and is a discerner of the thoughts and intents of the heart.
Hebrews 4:12, NKJV

For all the promises of God in Him are Yes, and in Him Amen, to the glory of God through us.
2 Corinthians 1:20, NKJV

Let's keep a firm grip on the promises that keep us going. He always keeps his word.
Hebrews 10: 23, MESSAGE

Now faith is the substance of things hoped for, the evidence of things not seen.
Hebrews 11:1, KJV

During the fourth watch of the night Jesus went out to them, walking on the lake. When the disciples saw him walking on the lake, they were terrified. "It's a ghost," they said, and cried out in fear.

But Jesus immediately said to them: "Take courage! It is I. Don't be afraid."

"Lord, if it's you," Peter replied, "tell me to come to you on the water."

"Come," he said.

Then Peter got down out of the boat, walked on the water and came toward Jesus. But when he saw the wind, he was afraid and, beginning to sink, cried out, "Lord, save me!"

Immediately Jesus reached out his hand and caught him. "You of little faith," he said, "why did you doubt?"
Matthew 14:25–31, NIV

Looking unto Jesus the author and finisher of our faith; who for the joy that was set before him endured the cross, despising the shame, and is set down at the right hand of the throne of God.
Hebrews 12:2, KJV

"It is finished." With that, he bowed his head and gave up his spirit.
John 19:30, NIV

The reason the Son of God appeared was to destroy the devil's work.
1 John 3:8, NIV

Every good and perfect gift is from above, coming down from the Father of heavenly lights, who does not change like shifting shadows.
James 1:17, NIV

The thief does not come except to steal, and to kill, and to destroy. I have come that they may have life, and that they may have it more abundantly.
John 10:10, NKJV

Is this the kind of fast I have chosen,
only a day for a man to humble himself?
Is it only for bowing one's head like a reed
and for lying on sackcloth and ashes?
Is that what you call a fast,
a day acceptable to the Lord ?
Is not this the kind of fasting I have chosen:
to loose the chains of injustice
and untie the cords of the yoke,
to set the oppressed free
and break every yoke?
Is it not to share your food with the hungry
and to provide the poor wanderer with shelter—
when you see the naked, to clothe him,
and not to turn away from your own flesh and blood?
Then your light will break forth like the dawn,
and your healing will quickly appear;
then your righteousness will go before you,
and the glory of the Lord will be your rear guard.
Then you will call, and the Lord will answer;
you will cry for help, and he will say: Here am I.
Isaiah 58:5–9, NIV

(To read the complete chapter of Isaiah 58, see a Bible.)

"The Year of the Lord's Favor"
The Spirit of the Sovereign Lord is on me,
because the Lord has anointed me
to preach good news to the poor.
He has sent me to bind up the brokenhearted,
to proclaim freedom for the captives
and release from darkness for the prisoners,
to proclaim the year of the Lord's favor
and the day of vengeance of our God,
to comfort all who mourn,

and provide for those who grieve in Zion—
to bestow on them a crown of beauty
instead of ashes,
the oil of gladness
instead of mourning,
and a garment of praise
instead of a spirit of despair.
Isaiah 61:1-3, NIV

(To read the complete chapter of Isaiah 68, see a Bible.)

God "has saved us and called us to a holy life—not because of anything we have done but because of his own purpose and grace. This grace was given us in Christ Jesus before the beginning of time."
2 Timothy 2:9, NIV

Being confident of this, that he who began a good work in you will carry it on to completion until the day of Christ Jesus.
Philippians 1:6, NIV

Neither height nor depth, nor anything else in all creation, will be able to separate us from the love of God that is in Christ Jesus our Lord.
Romans 8:39, NIV

For our struggle is not against flesh and blood, but against the rulers, against the authorities, against the powers of this dark world and against the spiritual forces of evil in the heavenly realms.
Ephesians 6:12, NIV

I say then: Walk in the Spirit, and you shall not fulfill the lust of the flesh. For the flesh lusts against the Spirit, and the Spirit against the flesh; and these are contrary to one another, so that you do not do the things that you wish.
Galatians 5:16-17, NKJV

Now the works of the flesh are evident, which are: adultery, fornication, uncleanness, lewdness, idolatry, sorcery, hatred, contentions, jealousies, outbursts of wrath, selfish ambitions, dissensions, heresies, 21envy, murders, drunkenness, revelries, and the like; of which I tell you beforehand, just as I also told you in time past, that those who practice such things will not inherit the kingdom of God.
Galatians 5:19-21, NKJV

Do not love the world or anything in the world. If anyone loves the world, the love of the Father is not in him. For everything in the world—the cravings of sinful man, the lust of his eyes and the boasting of what he has and does—comes not form the Father but from the world. The world and its desires pass away, but the man who does the will of God lives forever.
1 John 2:15-17, NIV

You belong to your father, the devil, and you want to carry out your father's desire.
He was a murderer from the beginning, not holding to the truth, for there is no truth in
him. When he lies, he speaks his native language, for he is a liar and the father
of lies.
John 8:44, NIV

No one can serve two masters. Either he will hate the one and love the other, or he will
be devoted to the one and despise the other. You cannot serve both God and Money.
Matthew 6:24, NIV

I have seen all the works that are done under the sun; and, behold, all is vanity and
vexation of spirit.
Ecclesiastes 1:14, KJV

Greater is he that is in you, than he that is in the world.
1 John 4:4, KJV

For what I do is not the good I want to do; no, the evil I do not want to do—this I keep
on doing.
Romans 7:19, NIV

That which is born of the flesh is flesh, and that which is born of the Spirit is spirit.
John 3:6, NIV

CHAPTER 3: THE ROOT OF IT ALL
WHAT'S BEHIND THIS ADDICTION?

He has sent me to bind up the brokenhearted, to proclaim freedom for the captives
and to release from darkness the prisoners.
Isaiah 61:1, NIV

The Lord, the Lord, the compassionate and gracious God, slow to anger, abounding
in love and faithfulness, maintaining love to thousands, and forgiving wickedness,
rebellion and sin. Yet he does not leave the guilty unpunished; he punishes the
children and their children for the sin of the fathers to the third and fourth generation.
Exodus 34:6-7, NIV

But the fruit of the Spirit is love, joy, peace, patience, kindness, goodness, faithfulness,
gentleness and self-control. Against such things there is no law.
Galatians 5:22-23, NIV

He chose to be mistreated along with the people of God rather than to enjoy the
pleasures of sin for a short time.
Hebrews 11:25, NIV

Pharaoh summoned Moses and Aaron and said, "Pray to the Lord to take the frogs away from me and my people, and I will let your people go to offer sacrifices to the Lord"

Moses said to Pharaoh, "I leave to you the honor of setting the time for me to pray for you and your officials and your people that you and your houses may be rid of the frogs, except for those that remain in the Nile."

"Tomorrow," Pharaoh said.
Exodus 8:8–10, NIV

CHAPTER 4: OUT WITH THE OLD AND IN WITH THE NEW

Therefore, there is now no condemnation for those who are in Christ Jesus, because through Christ Jesus the law of the Spirit of life set *me* free from the law of sin and death.
Romans 8:1–2, NIV *(italics added)*

So if the Son [Jesus] sets you free, you will be free indeed.
John 8:36, NIV

For we know that our old self was crucified with him so that the body of sin might be rendered powerless, that we should no longer be slaves to sin.
Romans 6:6, NIV

It shall come to pass in that day that his burden will be taken away from your shoulder, and his yoke from your neck, and the yoke will be destroyed because of the anointing.
Isaiah 10:27, NJKV

I will give them an undivided heart and put a new spirit in them; I will remove from them their heart of stone and give them a heart of flesh.
Ezekiel 11:19, NIV

For the word of God is living and active. Sharper than any double-edged sword, it penetrates even to dividing soul and spirit, joints and marrow; it judges the thoughts and attitudes of the heart.
Hebrews 4:12, NIV

The Spirit gives life; the flesh counts for nothing. The words I have spoken to you are spirit and they are life.
John 6:63, NIV

Heaven and earth will pass away, but my words will never pass away.
Mark 13:31, NIV

I tell you the truth, if anyone says to this mountain, "Go, throw yourself into the sea," and does not doubt in his heart but believes that what he says will happen, it will be done for him.
Mark 11:23, NIV

If we confess our sins, he is faithful and just and will forgive us our sins and purify us from all unrighteousness.
1 John 1:9, NIV

Repent, then, and turn to God, so that your sins may be wiped out, that times of refreshing may come from the Lord.
Acts 3:19, NIV

He who does what is sinful is of the devil, because the devil has been sinning from the beginning. The reason the Son of God appeared was to destroy the devil's work.
1 John 3:8, NIV

I know both how to be abased, and I know how to abound: every where and in all things I am instructed both to be full and to be hungry, both to abound and to suffer need. I can do all things through Christ which strengtheneth me.
Philippians 4:12–13, KJV

But he said to me, "My grace is sufficient for you, for my power is made perfect in weakness." Therefore I will boast all the more gladly about my weaknesses, so that Christ's power may rest on me.
2 Corinthians 12:9, NIV

Do not judge, and you will not be judged. Do not condemn, and you will not be condemned. Forgive, and you will be forgiven.
Luke 6:37, NIV

See to it that no one misses the grace of God and that no bitter root grows up to cause trouble and defile many.
Hebrews 12:15, NIV

"Forgive us our debts, as we also have forgiven our debtors. And lead us not into temptation, but deliver us from the evil one." For if you forgive men when they sin against you, your heavenly Father will also forgive you. But if you do not forgive men their sins, your Father will not forgive your sins.
Matthew 6:12–15, NIV

CHAPTER 5: WALKING IN FREEDOM, RESTORATION, AND HEALING

Examine yourselves to see whether you are in faith; test yourselves. Do you not realize that Christ Jesus is in you—unless, of course, you fail the test?
2 Corinthians 13:5, NIV

We're rooting for the truth to win out in you.
2 Corinthians 13:8, MESSAGE

In the same way, count yourselves dead to sin but alive to God in Christ Jesus.
Romans 6:11, NIV

I tell you the truth, whoever hears my word and believes him who sent me has eternal life and will not be condemned; he has crossed over from death to life.
John 5:24, NIV

The Parable of the Lost Son

Jesus continued: "There was a man who had two sons. The younger one said to his father, 'Father, give me my share of the estate.' So he divided his property between them.

"Not long after that, the younger son got together all he had, set off for a distant country and there squandered his wealth in wild living. After he had spent everything, there was a severe famine in that whole country, and he began to be in need. So he went and hired himself out to a citizen of that country, who sent him to his fields to feed pigs. He longed to fill his stomach with the pods that the pigs were eating, but no one gave him anything.

"When he came to his senses, he said, 'How many of my father's hired men have food to spare, and here I am starving to death! I will set out and go back to my father and say to him: Father, I have sinned against heaven and against you. I am no longer worthy to be called your son; make me like one of your hired men.' So he got up and went to his father.
"But while he was still a long way off, his father saw him and was filled with compassion for him; he ran to his son, threw his arms around him and kissed him.

"The son said to him, 'Father, I have sinned against heaven and against you. I am no longer worthy to be called your son.'

"But the father said to his servants, 'Quick! Bring the best robe and put it on him. Put a ring on his finger and sandals on his feet. Bring the fattened calf and kill it. Let's have a feast and celebrate. For this son of mine was dead and is alive again; he was lost and is found.' So they began to celebrate.

"Meanwhile, the older son was in the field. When he came near the house, he heard music and dancing. So he called one of the servants and asked him what was going on. 'Your brother has come,' he replied, 'and your father has killed the fattened calf because he has him back safe and sound.'

"The older brother became angry and refused to go in. So his father went out and pleaded with him. But he answered his father, 'Look! All these years I've been slaving for you and never disobeyed your orders. Yet you never gave me even a young goat so I could celebrate with my friends. But when this son of yours who has squandered your property with prostitutes comes home, you kill the fattened calf for him!'

"'My son,' the father said, 'you are always with me, and everything I have is yours. But we had to celebrate and be glad, because this brother of yours was dead and is alive again; he was lost and is found.'"

Luke 15:11–32, NIV

Therefore I tell you, whatever you ask for in prayer, believe that you have received it, and it will be yours.
Mark 11:24, NIV

"Is not my word like fire," says the Lord, "and like a hammer that breaks a rock in pieces?"
Jeremiah 23:29, NIV

So if the Son sets you free, you will be free indeed.
John 8:36, NIV

Submit yourselves, then, to God. Resist the devil, and he will flee from you.
James 4:7, NIV

No temptation has seized you except what is common to man. And God is faithful; he will not let you be tempted beyond what you can bear. But when you are tempted, he will also provide a way out so that you can stand up under it.
1 Corinthians 10:13, NIV *(italics added)*

Stand fast therefore in the liberty wherewith Christ hath made us free, and be not entangled again with the yoke of bondage.
Galatians 5:1, KJV

You, dear children, are from God and have overcome them, because the one who is in you is greater than the one who is in the world.
1 John 4:4, NIV

For no matter how many promises God has made, they are "Yes" in Christ. And so through him the "Amen" is spoken by us to the glory of God.
2 Corinthians 1:20, NIV

They overcame him by the blood of the Lamb and by the word of their testimony; they did not love their lives so much as to shrink from death.
Revelation 12:11, NIV

Jesus answered, "It is written: 'Man does not live on bread alone, but on every word that comes from the mouth of God.'" . . . Jesus answered him, It is also written: Do

not put the Lord your God to the test. . . . Jesus said to him, Away from me, satan! For it is written: Worship the Lord your God, and serve him only.
Matthew 4:4, 7, 10, NIV

So is my word that goes out from my mouth: It will not return to me empty, but will accomplish what I desire and achieve the purpose for which I sent it.
Isaiah 55:11, NIV

The king was overjoyed and gave orders to lift Daniel out of the den. And when Daniel was lifted from the den, no wound was found on him, because he had trusted in his God.
Daniel 6:23, NIV

The end of all things is near. Therefore be clear minded and self-controlled so that you can pray.
1 Peter 4:7, NIV

Whom having not seen, ye love; in whom, though now ye see him not, yet believing, ye rejoice with joy unspeakable and full of glory.
1 Peter 1:8, KJV

You have made known to me the path of life; you will fill me with joy in your presence, with eternal pleasures at your right hand.
Psalm 16:11, NIV

Nehemiah said, "Go and enjoy choice food and sweet drinks, and send some to those who have nothing prepared. This day is sacred to our Lord. Do not grieve, for the joy of the LORD is your strength."
Nehemiah 8:10, NIV

A cheerful heart is good medicine, but a crushed spirit dries up the bones.
Proverbs 17:22, NIV

But encourage one another daily, as long as it is called Today, so that none of you may be hardened by sin's deceitfulness.
Hebrews 3:13, NIV

(To read Psalm 100 in its entirety, see a Bible.)

Shout for joy to the Lord, all the earth.

Worship the Lord with gladness;
come before him with joyful songs.
Know that the Lord is God.
It is he who made us, and we are his;
we are his people, the sheep of his pasture.
Enter his gates with thanksgiving
and his courts with praise;
give thanks to him and praise his name.
For the Lord is good and his love endures forever;
his faithfulness continues through all generations.
From the lips of children and infants
you have ordained praise
because of your enemies,
to silence the foe and the avenger.
Psalm 8:2, NIV

But thou art holy, O thou that inhabitest the praises of Israel.
Psalm 22:3, KJV

After consulting the people, Jehoshaphat appointed men to sing to the Lord and to praise him for the splendor of his holiness as they went out at the head of the army, saying:

"Give thanks to the Lord,

for his love endures forever."

As they began to sing and praise, the Lord set ambushes against the men of Ammon and Moab and Mount Seir who were invading Judah, and they were defeated.

2 Chronicles 20:21-22, NIV

What this means is that those who become Christians become new persons. They are not the same anymore, for the old life is gone. A new life has begun!
2 Corinthians 5:17, NLT

Run from anything that stimulates youthful lust. Follow anything that makes you want to do right. Pursue faith and love and peace, and enjoy the companionship of those who call on the Lord with pure hearts.
2 Timothy 2:22, NLT

The thief cometh not, but for to steal, and to kill, and to destroy: I am come that they might have life, and that they might have it more abundantly.
John 10:10, KJV

As it is written: "I have made you a father of many nations." He is our father in the sight of God, in whom he believed—the God who gives life to the dead and calls things that are not as though they were.
Romans 4:17, NIV

But he was wounded and crushed for our sins. He was beaten that we might have peace. He was whipped, and we were healed!
Isaiah 53:5, NLT

Who his own self bare our sins in his own body on the tree, that we, being dead to sins, should live unto righteousness: by whose stripes ye were healed.
1 Peter 2:24, KJV

CHAPTER 6: BIG GOD—BIG FREE
FREE TO FIGHT FOR OTHERS AND FOLLOW GOD

Praise be to the God and Father of our Lord Jesus Christ, the Father of compassion and the God of all comfort, who comforts us in all our troubles, so that we can comfort those in any trouble with the comfort we ourselves have received from God.
2 Corinthians 1:3-4, NIV

He has made us competent as ministers of a new covenant—not of the letter [of the law] but of the Spirit, for the letter kills, but the Spirit gives life.
2 Corinthians 3:6, NIV

By the power of signs and miracles, through the power of the Spirit. So from Jerusalem all the way around to Illyricum, I have fully proclaimed the gospel of Christ.
Romans 15:19, NIV

For [although] they hold a form of piety (true religion), they deny and reject and are strangers to the power of it [their conduct belies the genuineness of their profession]. Avoid [all] such people [turn away from them].
2 Timothy 3:5, AMPLIFIED

For bodily exercise profits a little, but godliness is profitable for all things, having promise of the life that now is and of that which is to come.
1 Timothy 4:8, NKJV

If you really knew me, you would know my Father as well. From now on, you do know him and have seen him.
John 14:7, NIV

Not that I have already obtained all this, or have already been made perfect, but I press on to take hold of that for which Christ Jesus took hold of me.
Philippians 3:12, NIV

"For I know the plans I have for you," declares the Lord, "plans to prosper you and not to harm you, plans to give you hope and a future."
Jeremiah 29:11, NIV

Being confident of this, that he who began a good work in you will carry it on to completion until the day of Christ Jesus.
Philippians 1:6, NIV

Do you not know that in a race all the runners run, but only one gets the prize? Run in such a way as to get the prize.
1 Corinthians 9:24, NIV

Blessed is the man who perseveres under trial, because when he has stood the test, he will receive the crown of life that God has promised to those who love him.
James 1:12, NIV

Do not be afraid of what you are about to suffer. I tell you, the devil will put some of you in prison to test you, and you will suffer persecution for ten days. Be faithful, even to the point of death, and I will give you the crown of life. He who has an ear, let him hear what the Spirit says to the churches. He who overcomes will not be hurt at all by the second death.
Revelation 2:10–11, NIV

The entrance of Your words gives light; it gives understanding to the simple.
Psalm 119:130, NKJV

I pray that out of his glorious riches he may strengthen you with power through his Spirit in your inner being, so that Christ may dwell in your hearts through faith. And I pray that you, being rooted and established in love, may have power . . . to grasp how wide and long and high and deep is the love of Christ, and to know this love that surpasses knowledge that you may be filled to the measure of all the fullness of God.
Ephesians 3:16–19, NIV

CHAPTER 7: FAQS AND A LIBERTY TOOL KIT

"Frequently Asked Questions" Scriptures

And Peter opened his mouth and said: Most certainly and thoroughly I now perceive and understand that God shows no partiality and is no respecter of persons.
Acts 10:34, AMPLIFIED

Thus you nullify the word of God for the sake of your tradition.
Matthew 15:6, NIV

Teach me to do your will, for you are my God. May your gracious Spirit lead me forward on a firm footing.
Psalm 143:10, NLT

(To read John chapter 16 and Acts chapters 1, 2, 8, and 1, see a Bible.)

We demolish arguments and every pretension that sets itself up against the knowledge of God, and we take captive every thought to make it obedient to Christ.
2 Corinthians 10:5, NIV

(To read Jude see a Bible.)

"Making Jesus Your Lord and Savior" Scriptures

And everyone who calls on the name of the Lord will be saved.
Acts 2:21, NIV

That if you confess with your mouth, "Jesus is Lord," and believe in your heart that God raised him from the dead, you will be saved. For it is with your heart that you believe and are justified, and it is with your mouth that you confess and are saved. As the Scripture says, "Anyone who trusts in him will never be put to shame." For there is no difference between Jew and Gentile—the same Lord is Lord of all and richly blesses all who call on him, for, "Everyone who calls on the name of the Lord will be saved."
Romans 10:9-13, NIV

For God so loved the world that he gave his one and only Son, that whoever believes in him shall not perish but have eternal life.
John 3:16, NIV

All that the Father gives me will come to me, and whoever comes to me I will never drive away.
John 6:37 NIV

"Immersion in the Holy Spirit and Speaking in Spiritual Tongues" Scriptures

If you then, though you are evil, know how to give good gifts to your children, how much more will your Father in heaven give the Holy Spirit to those who ask him!
Luke 11:13, NIV

All of them were filled with the Holy Spirit and began to speak in other tongues as the Spirit enabled them.
Acts 2:4, NIV

And I will ask the Father, and he will give you another Counselor to be with you forever—the Spirit of truth. The world cannot accept him, because it neither sees him nor knows him. But you know him, for he lives with you and will be in you
John 14:16-17, NIV

However, as it is written: "No eye has seen, no ear has heard, no mind has conceived what God has prepared for those who love him"—but God has revealed it to us by his Spirit.

The Spirit searches all things, even the deep things of God. For who among men knows the thoughts of a man except the man's spirit within him? In the same way no one knows the thoughts of God except the Spirit of God. We have not received the spirit of the world but the Spirit who is from God, that we may understand what God has freely given us. This is what we speak, not in words taught us by human wisdom but in words taught by the Spirit, expressing spiritual truths in spiritual words.

1 Corinthians 2:9–13, NIV

In the same way, the Spirit helps us in our weakness. We do not know what we ought to pray for, but the Spirit himself intercedes for us with groans that words cannot express.
Romans 8:26, NIV

But you, dear friends, build yourselves up in your most holy faith and pray in the Holy Spirit.
Jude 20, NIV

See also: *Luke 24:49; Eph. 3:19; 5:18-19; 6:18; Acts 1:4-8; 1st Cor. 14; & Mark 16:17*

Proclamation Card Scriptures

So if the Son sets you free, you will be free indeed.
John 8:36, NIV

But when the time had fully come, God sent his Son, born of a woman, born under law, to redeem those under law, that we might receive the full rights of sons.
Galatians 4:4–5, NIV

For God so loved the world that He gave His only begotten Son, that whoever believes in Him should not perish but have everlasting life. For God did not send His Son into the world to condemn the world, but that the world through Him might be saved.
John 3:16–17, NKJV

How great is the love the Father has lavished on us, that we should be called children of God! And that is what we are! . . .
1 John 3:1, NIV

Therefore, there is now no condemnation for those who are in Christ Jesus, because through Christ Jesus the law of the Spirit of life set me free from the law of sin and death.
Romans 8:1–2, NIV

Don't you know that you yourselves are God's temple and that God's Spirit lives in you?
1 Corinthians 3:16, NIV

And everyone who has this hope in Him [Jesus] purifies himself, just as He is pure.
1 John 3:3, NKJV

Examine yourselves to see whether you are in faith; test yourselves. Do you not realize that Christ Jesus is in you—unless, of course, you fail the test?
2 Corinthians 13:5, NIV

I tell you the truth, whatever you bind on earth will be bound in heaven, and whatever you loose on earth will be loosed in heaven.
Matthew 18:18, NIV

In the same way, count yourselves dead to sin but alive to God in Christ Jesus.
Romans 6:11, NIV

Greater is he that is in you, than he that is in the world.
1 John 4:4, KJV

Submit yourselves, then, to God. Resist the devil, and he will flee from you.
James 4:7, NIV

For all the promises of God in Him are Yes, and in Him Amen, to the glory of God through us.
2 Corinthians 1:20, NKJV

Stand fast therefore in the liberty wherewith Christ hath made us free, and be not entangled again with the yoke of bondage.
Galatians 5:1, KJV

Who his own self bare our sins in his own body on the tree, that we, being dead to sins, should live unto righteousness: by whose stripes ye were healed.
1 Peter 2:24, KJV

For I know the plans I have for you," declares the Lord, "plans to prosper you and not to harm you, plans to give you hope and a future."
Jeremiah 29:11, NIV

Being confident of this, that he who began a good work in you will carry it on to completion until the day of Christ Jesus.
Philippians 1:6, NIV

Do you not know that in a race all the runners run, but only one gets the prize? Run in such a way as to get the prize.
1 Corinthians 9:24, NIV

Do not be afraid of what you are about to suffer. I tell you, the devil will put some of you in prison to test you, and you will suffer persecution for ten days. Be faithful, even to the point of death, and I will give you the crown of life. He who has an ear, let him hear what the Spirit says to the churches. He who overcomes will not be hurt at all by the second death.
Revelation 2:10–11, NIV

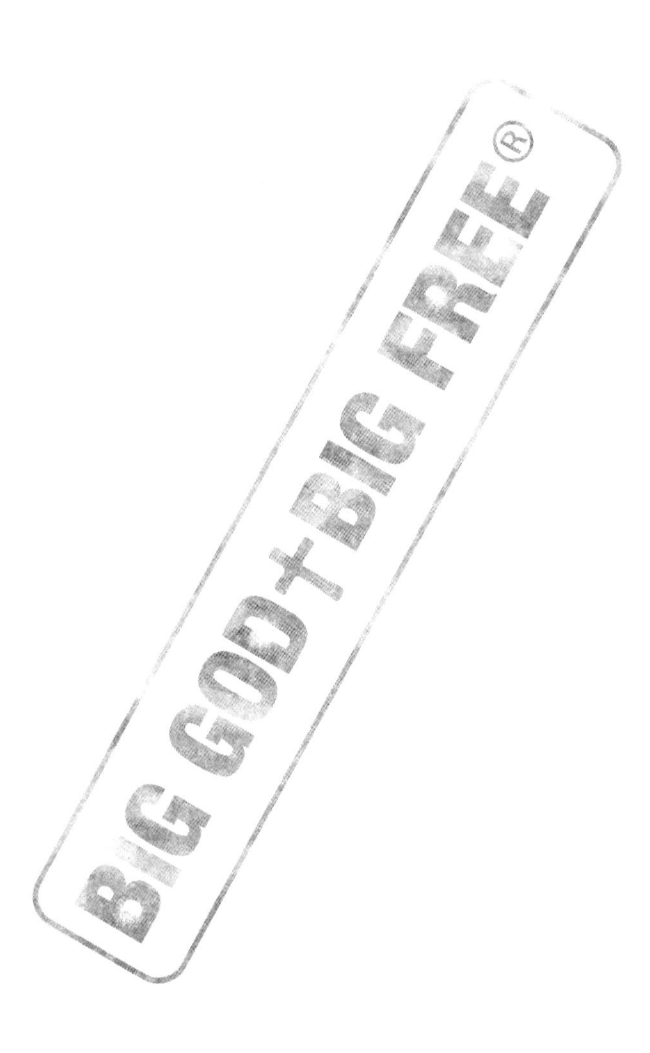

BIG GOD†BIG FREE®

BIBLIOGRAPHY

ARTICLES:

Covey, Stephen. (1991, November) Seven habits revisited: seven unique human endowments. Retrieved November 8, 2004, from http:// franklincovey.com/foryou/articles/seven.html

BOOKS:

Wigglesworth, Smith (2000)—Experiencing God's Power Today. Pennsylvania: Whitaker House.

TEACHINGS:

Allum, Isabel (2005)—Kingdom Identity. Spoken at the Grand River Church April 2, 2005, Grand Rapids, Michigan.

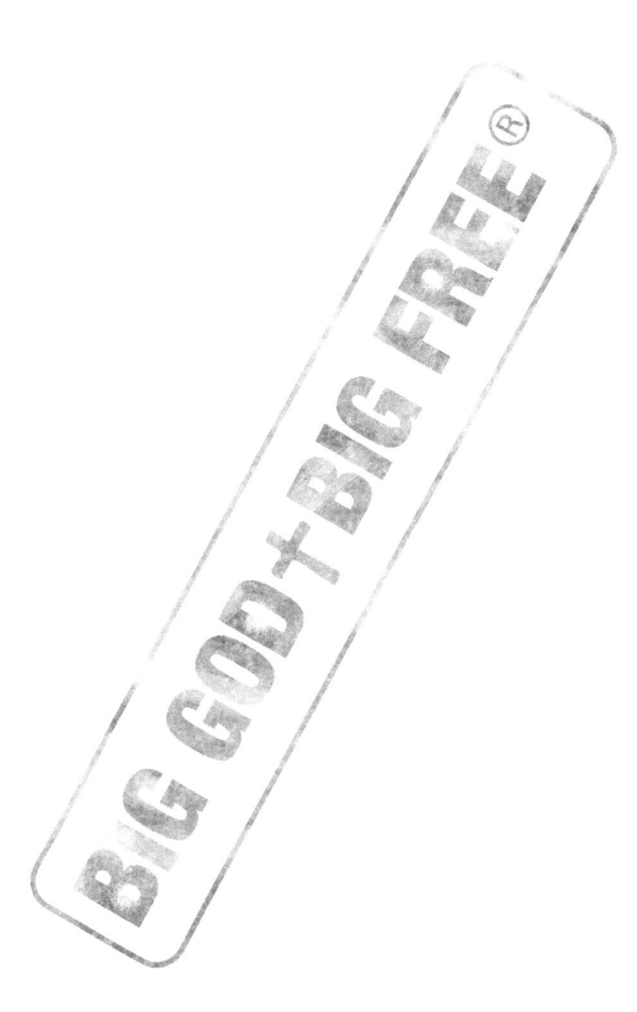

BIG GOD†BIG FREE®

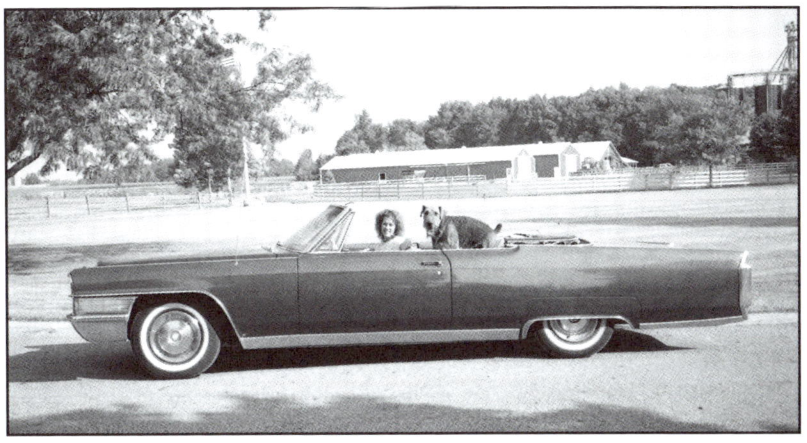

MICHELLE'S BIO

INTRODUCTION:

Michelle Behrenwald is an entrepreneur and blood bought child of God living in the United States. She believes God is a Big God who wants His children to live abundantly in freedom. God has proven that He's bigger than anything that has tried to tie her up or keep her down. As you can see, she is into Big – Big God, big car and big dog! "Before I become a sold-out child of God, she said, "I was confused because most people's rendition of God wasn't very big – all I ever wanted was to know God for who He really is – Omni everything and He is – plus He loves me unconditionally and immeasurably! He is bigger than anything I bring to Him." In fact, she calls herself a "Designer Original signed by God™", and she is passionate about others knowing and understanding that they, too, are the Creator's one-of-a-kind designer originals. "Each of us has a high calling, divine purpose and place, which only God can give us – "only let the Lord God Almighty define you – nobody else!"

BACKGROUND:

Michelle holds a Masters Degree in Communications, and her experience includes over twenty years as a global business executive, a university instructor and an auctioneer. Michelle is also the founder of by desiGn ministries, inc., which exists to help restore and free people and to encourage them as they follow God. She focuses on pioneering biblically based ministries which use "God's Truth" to solve social issues. She teaches a "Free Indeed" series that helps people get set free from any hindrances like addictions, fear, anxiety, anger, stress or generational curses so that they can walk forward into God's blessings, freedom and divine purpose for their lives.

Michelle is surrounded by her animal entourage and she enjoys the great outdoors, which daily reminds her of God's wondrous creativity. Encouraging others to grow and develop strong relationships with God and each other, while inspiring a sense of God's wonder and awe through nature, is part of her life's work. Michelle enjoys traveling the world and working with the Lord—ministering God's love and freedom to people everywhere.

TESTIMONY:

I'm an "overcomer" myself, freed from lots of things, addictions, fears, guilt, anger, pain and shame. When you live life, you receive a lot of damage—and sometimes when we are damaged; we become something we don't want to be. But Good News, God has provided a way out in Jesus Christ. I am a living testament to God's Way. I want to get freer everyday. My goal is that I can walk out my front door and no matter what happens that day, it will not effect me because of whose I am and His unconditional love for me. That doesn't mean life won't have its humps and bumps, it sure will, it is a fallen world we live in. The devil and his forces are always trying to seduce you and contest your liberty, but with Jesus Christ in you and the Holy Spirit as your helper, you go through it differently. With Jesus on your side, you have a love and a blood covering.

There is nothing to fear in life, for God will never leave you nor forsake you. I know, He is no respecter of persons and what He has done for me, He will do for you. He loves you. He made you. He signed you like a work of art. He paid the price for you and He loves you. Nothing can separate you from God's love. He is more than able. He is a Big Big God —bigger than anything you bring His way—bigger than any enemy —His love can go deeper than any wound the enemy has made in you. So go on—get free—Freedom in Jesus!

Be blessed—stick with God and see you in heaven someday!

Michelle

BIG GOD ✝ BIG FREE®

Interested in additional resources and materials *(Encouragement Audio Clips, Ministry Teachings, Prayers, & Humorous Reflections)* to assist you and others in your freedom walk?

Check out our website below:

www.BigGodBigFree.com

STAY THE COURSE
KEEP GETTING FREE!